Clinical Ambulatory Anesthesia

Clinical Ambulatory Anesthesia

Johan Raeder

Director of Ambulatory Anesthesia, Oslo University Hospital and Professor of Anesthesiology, University of Oslo, Norway

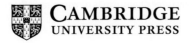

CAMBRIDGE UNIVERSITY PRESS

CAMBRIDGE UNIVERSITY PRESS
Cambridge, New York, Melbourne, Madrid, Cape Town, Singapore,
São Paulo, Delhi, Dubai, Tokyo

Cambridge University Press
The Edinburgh Building, Cambridge CB2 8RU, UK

Published in the United States of America by Cambridge University Press, New York

www.cambridge.org
Information on this title: www.cambridge.org/9780521737814

First published 2010

Printed in the United Kingdom at the University Press, Cambridge

A catalog record for this publication is available from the British Library

ISBN 978-0-521-73781-4 Paperback

Contents

Preface

My ambition with this book is to provide a guide to applied and practical ways of achieving ambulatory anesthesia. Ambulatory anesthesia incorporates most anesthetic topics and knowledge, but the focus is shifted somewhat from looking solely at what happens in the operating room to viewing the complete perioperative period. Although safety and quality in the operating room remain major goals, the ambulatory anesthetist should always plan to optimize the postoperative period. This is not an exhaustive textbook, but rather a selection of topics that I think are important in this context for the anesthesiologist. I have also incorporated brief surveys on important aspects of organization, unit setup, and quality assurance, as the anesthesiologist often will be the perioperative physician involved through-out the patient's treatment, from start to finish. Discussions of and references to basic anesthesiological knowledge should be sought elsewhere, but I hope to bring forward some issues related to, and evidence for, the pragmatic and good practice of ambulatory anesthesia. However, in many cases there is no firm evidence or there is conflicting evidence regarding different aspects of the case. As anesthetists must make decisions under these circumstances, I have tried to guide you based on more than 25 years of clinical practice in most kinds of ambulatory and office-based practice. I have also tried to incorporate knowledge from our own clinical research as well as the research and teaching by my many good friends working on the international ambulatory anesthesia scene. Special thanks are due to my two good friends Professor Kari Korttila, who introduced me to the international organization of ambulatory anesthesia, and Professor Paul F. White, who has nourished me over many years with his vast personal knowledge. I also wish to express my gratitude to everyone who has worked with me over the years, for all their unceasing inspiration and good ideas. Further, I gratefully acknowledge my supportive family and Cambridge University Press for providing me with all help and this great opportunity.

Johan Raeder
Oslo

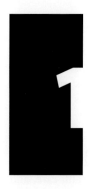

Background to ambulatory surgery and anesthesia

Definitions [1]

The formal distinction between *inpatient*, *ambulatory*, and *outpatient* is quite important to make, although the medical approach will be dictated by the patient, the planned surgical procedure, and the context. This has to do with benchmarking, statistics, finances, and formal rules; as well as defining levels of care with different levels of resource allocation expected.

The International Association of Ambulatory Surgery (IAAS) defines *ambulatory surgery* as: "An operation/procedure, excluding an office or outpatient operation/procedure, where the patient is discharged on the same working day" (http://iaas-med.com/modules/content/ Acr977.tmp.pdf), in contrast to inpatient surgery where the patients stay in hospital overnight. Although the American definition, because of old rules of insurance companies and systems of payment, allows for 23-h stays to be classed as ambulatory this does not seem to be a fruitful concept. The whole idea with ambulatory surgery is to have the patient ready for discharge to a setting without health care staffing within the scope of a single working day, basically with the same team of carers involved during all or most of the session. Sessions may be designated as morning, afternoon, or evening, and sometimes overlap between these sessions is required, but whatever the case the fundamental and very simple end point for ambulatory care is that the patient does not spend the night in a staffed health care institution. Hotel or hospital-hotel stay can be classed as ambulatory as long as there are no dedicated health personnel there to routinely look after the patient. Having a backup service if needed, such as a receptionist or even a nurse when requested, falls within the ambulatory concept; the point is that these carers will not look after the patient unless called for by the patient or their chaperone.

The distinction of ambulatory surgery from a simple *outpatient consultation* entailing some procedures is more challenging and not that straightforward to make. Most will agree that all procedures requiring general anesthesia should be classified as ambulatory, including those procedures that are usually done under a general but in some cases can be carried out using regional or local anesthesia or sedation, or a combination of these options. Still there are areas of potential dispute, as the following examples show. Where is the outpatient/ambulatory distinction between a simple scar correction and an extensive plastic surgical procedure where both are carried out under local anesthesia? Diagnostic rectoscopy versus removal of a rectal tumor by a rectoscope? The removal of stitches from a wound versus removal of screws from a bone?

A pragmatic and useful distinction is to designate cases as outpatient when the patient is generally expected not to need any specialized care or specialized surveillance when the procedure is finished. Using this approach an endoscopy (cystoscopy, gastroscopy, colonoscopy) should not be considered ambulatory unless general anesthesia is used or an intervention (e.g., tumor removal) is required necessitating post-procedural observation in a health care facility in case of bleeding or other complications. Similarly, most procedures carried out using regional anesthesia or deep sedation should be classified as ambulatory where some post-procedural professional observation is required.

Short history of ambulatory surgery and anesthesia [2]

Going back only 200 years presents us with a totally different scenario of health care, and especially surgery, compared with today. The average life expectancy was about 40–50 years, there were no effective painkillers, no antibiotics and hardly any efficient drugs as such, although some herbs with therapeutic potential were in use. Surgery had a very high mortality, the patient dying from cardiovascular stress with unbearable pain during the procedure, from bleeding (there was no intravenous technology available), or from wound infection escalating to sepsis or necrosis (no knowledge about hygiene and sterility; no antibiotics). Nowadays on average about 1 in 10 people have a surgical procedure every year in the developed world, whereas 200 years ago the figure was about 1 out of 2 000–5 000 people. The very few cases done were either quite minor or quick, such as removal of foreign bodies, reposition of fractures, puncture of abscesses, etc., or they were occasionally carried out to treat clearly life-threatening conditions, for example a skull burr hole for extradural hematoma evacuation. The procedures were undertaken in the patient's home or in the field. The first hospitals were built in the time of war near battlefields where it seemed practical to assemble the large number of severely injured soldiers in dedicated tents, huts, or houses, basically for simple wound care and amputations. Some hospitals emerged in the cities as well, to offer services to the poor and homeless; the wealthy and nobility having their health care provided at home. The development of modern anesthesia occurred in the 1840s with ether anesthesia and nitrous oxide being major revolutions in the history of medicine. For the first time it became possible to undertake prolonged and complex surgical procedures on patients whose consciousness was controlled by ether vapor. By the end of the nineteenth century the technology of intravenous infusion and drugs had become available, and cocaine was introduced as the first example of a local anesthetic. Expansion in surgical techniques and technology together with development of sterile routines peroperatively led to a dramatic increase in the number of surgical procedures being undertaken. Many hospitals were built to accommodate the new era. By the beginning of the twentieth century the rule was for all surgery to be undertaken in hospital-like institutions, with patients staying in bed receiving nursing care for many days after the procedure. Even as late as 1960–1970 the general rule was for patients having a cholecystectomy to stay in hospital for at least 3–5 days and even those having a hernia repair stayed in for many days, even for 1–2 weeks in many places.

The modern ambulatory surgery era started just after 1900 with pioneering institutions in the USA and the UK, which had a hospital setup but sent patients home in the evening.

Later development was quite scattered, with pioneering institutions in many places, but it was not until 1970–1980 that ambulatory surgery became a forceful movement with an everyday impact on health care in the western world. Today, about 50–70% of all surgical procedures are ambulatory in the most highly developed countries, whereas the number in Eastern Europe, Africa, and most places in Asia and South America remains less than 5–10%. These percentages are always calculated in terms of procedure number, which is quite different from the "amount" of surgery, which is a term that also encompasses the total time, personnel, and resources spent on surgery. Obviously, because ambulatory surgery is not possible in major, prolonged, and emergent cases, the fraction of total surgical resources spent on ambulatory cases will be far less than 50–70%.

Why ambulatory surgery?

The usefulness of ambulatory surgery should be discussed in a context of looking at its pros and cons from perspectives of: (1) safety; (2) quality; (3) economics; and (4) education and staff satisfaction.

A pertinent question to ask is why do we send patients home on the same day of surgery in the most wealthy countries, which really could afford to provide an overnight service to their population? As this is a successful approach and accepted by the population, it is probably conceived as being safe and carrying the appropriate quality; otherwise this practice would have been hotly debated. A more complex follow-up question is why ambulatory surgery is not a major feature in less wealthy countries that could make savings by avoiding having many patients staying for days unnecessarily in staffed hospitals. This may be due to the prerequisites of successful ambulatory surgery as discussed in more detail in Chapter 2.

Ambulatory surgery requires an established infrastructure within the ambulatory unit and it is a disciplined and demanding process to change from inpatient to outpatient care. The personnel need to adopt new routines and tighter schedules, the patients need to be better informed, and the surgical and anesthesiological procedures need to be updated for same-day discharge to be feasible. The backup systems outside the hospital, such as phone access, road communication, ambulance systems, and well-informed chaperones, need to be adequate. Further, in most nonwealthy countries the unemployment rate is high and salaries for overnight nurses or carers are low, thus there may not be much incentive (maybe even some resistance) to close down these units during nights and weekends. Also, ambulatory care requires a health care financial system that acts as an incentive for those involved and not as a disincentive as is the case when hospital income is based on inpatient numbers. This is quite evident when looking at, for instance, Germany, where the fraction of ambulatory care was much lower than in other western countries until recently, when the reimbursement system was changed from a system with economic "punishment" of those who carried out ambulatory surgery.

A modern approach is to twist the question round and instead of asking whether a patient could go home and defining the criteria, one could ask, "Is there any reason why this patient should stay overnight?" Then criteria could be laid down for when an overnight stay is needed, based on defined reasons, for example safety, quality, or total economy. Another way of challenging the overnight stay dogma is to ask, "What will be different with inpatient care?" Frequently, "overnight stay" implies that the patient is sent to the ward late in the afternoon. Then patients may be left alone in their rooms for many hours consecutively during the night, unless otherwise requested. Again, questions should be asked about the potential worst-case scenario and issues of perceived quality; namely is the patient care best provided in the hospital or at home with a responsible escort?

Safety

In a study of more than 45 000 patients for 30 days after an ambulatory surgical procedure, Warner et al. concluded that the major morbidity (i.e., respiratory, circulatory, cardiac) was similar to that in the general population not having surgery [3]. In a more recent study of

18 500 Danish ambulatory surgical patients, there were no cases of death or permanent disability that could be ascribed to the procedure during a 90-day follow-up [4]. Some procedures have a relatively high risk, such as tonsillectomy, where a 1 in 10 000 mortality rate was reported in Norway over the last 5–10 years (Raeder, J., data on file), although these deaths were related to substandard care and not to the ambulatory concepts per se. Also, cases of inadvertent artery puncture or gut puncture with peritonitis have been reported with laparoscopy, but, again, these are not related to the ambulatory setting. In a study of ambulatory liposuction in Florida, Vila et al. found a tenfold increase in mortality when these procedures were performed in physicians' offices with improper standards, compared with licensed ambulatory centers [5].

We may conclude on some issues regarding safety in ambulatory care:

a. The safety is very close to 100% when proper ambulatory care is undertaken. This means the patient should feel safe but also that there is zero tolerance for serious errors in patient handling in the ambulatory setting.

b. Ambulatory surgery is safe because of good standards of care. If the standards are suboptimal, ambulatory surgery (as well as inpatient surgery) may not be safe and acceptable.

c. Some procedures will have a risk of rare and/or serious complications that is not avoided by doing the procedure in an ambulatory setting. Thus, care of ambulatory patients should be carried out using the same standards and resources as is care of inpatients.

Quality

There are a number of quality issues in favor of ambulatory care, which are listed below:

a. The risk of having a hospital infection is reduced as the patients are subjected less to the hospital environment, both in terms of exposure duration and also because ambulatory surgery is usually undertaken in premises with less contamination by seriously ill inpatients. In our own study the rate of infection after mixed ambulatory surgery during a 30-day observation period was 3.4%, being mostly benign, superficial wound infections [6]. The infection rate in comparable inpatients was in the range of 5–15%. Also in a study by Holtz and Wenzel the infection rate was about 3 times higher in inpatients when compared with ambulatory surgery [7].

b. Reversible cognitive dysfunction for some weeks or even months after surgery may be seen in up to 20–40% of the patients, more frequently with older age and extensive surgery [8]. The risk of cognitive dysfunction 1 week after hernia repair in elderly patients was significantly reduced from 9.8% with inpatient care to 3.8% (similar to nonoperated) after ambulatory care [9]. This seems logical: elderly patients especially, but also psychiatric patients, patients with cerebral dysfunction, and children, may all be stressed and confused by being subjected to an unfamiliar environment and unfamiliar people, and the longer the exposure the worse the effect. Thus, the sooner these types of patients can go safely back to their familiar environment, the better [10].

c. Less internal transport and fewer carers. This has to do with the shorter chain of treatment in ambulatory care; no wards are involved either pre- or postoperatively and most often the whole sequence from admission to discharge occurs in one area with the same personnel throughout. This increases continuity in terms of information provided and results in fewer misunderstandings. Also the information may be perceived as being better because the patient has to receive certain information before being discharged, whereas for inpatients the discharge process is often less consistent.

d. Less bed rest and immobility. The whole ambulatory setting is based on elective patients who are mobile and wearing their own clothes when they arrive and when they leave. They should be routinely seated in chairs and walk into theater themselves, unless unable to do so. This contrasts with the inpatient setting, where being in bed and bed rest are the default states. Being mobilized is good for many reasons: better gut function, better lung function, lower risk of thrombosis, and less chance of feeling ill.

e. Fewer delays and cancellations. The ambulatory surgical path is usually organized with its own nursing staff and dedicated facilities. The risk of a case being postponed because of an incidental burden from emergency care surgery or because there is no room in the postanesthesia care unit (PACU) is less than when minor procedures are done as inpatients between major surgery cases.

f. "Home is best." If you ask patients where they want to be after surgery provided that they are and feel safe, have no nausea and no or minor pain, most will prefer to be at home together with a spouse or friend than stay overnight in an unfamiliar hospital room.

Economy

It is beyond the scope of this book to discuss the economics of the ambulatory health care system in detail, but in brief it avoids expenses due to nursing care and patient accommodation in the late evening and overnight. The costs of doing the procedure, including all costs related to surgery and anesthesia, are the same as if the patient were an inpatient. Still, the situation may not be so simple. For a single hospital or unit to make such savings, the ambulatory program needs to be big enough to produce reduced staffing levels. Alternatively, the program needs to be large and predictable enough to release beds to other patients, thus increasing hospital production rather than saving money. In order for patients to have a rapid and uneventful recovery, more expensive anesthetic drugs may have to be used, but this expenditure may be recouped in reduced length of time in the operating room and reduced stay and need for nursing care in the PACU. It has also been shown in many places that focusing on ambulatory care results in the less dogmatic use of routine tests and associated savings, as most tests on ambulatory patients are done only for specific indications. The involvement of fewer carers reduces the need for handover between carers and reduces the extent of double documentation, which is often seen when many people are involved with one patient. Establishment of an ambulatory service may by itself improve the efficiency of the hospital, as a large amount of work occurs in a predictable manner with few cancellations and no interruptions by and disputes over emergency cases. A potential cost problem with ambulatory care is when very expensive equipment (e.g., laparoscopy racks, robots, etc.) is used only during the daytime; but this may be solved by have dedicated afternoon lists or by using the equipment in other places in the hospital when the ambulatory operating room is down. Ambulatory care may also be expensive if too many patients planned for ambulatory care have to be admitted unexpectedly, if they need a lot of expert care after being sent home, or if there is a high rate of unplanned readmission.

Education and staff satisfaction

Most staff will be happy to reduce the number of hours worked during evenings, nights, and weekends; thus recruitment and continuity in ambulatory care units are usually very good. However, there is some concern that ambulatory cases are too predictable and rarely present with emergencies and difficult situations. This may be overcome by having personnel rotate in and out of the unit for those who want to, and by having regular training in important emergency routines, such as advanced cardiorespiratory resuscitation. For the anesthesiologist it may be useful to have emergency praxis in between work at the ambulatory unit, or to attend training sessions or simulations in relevant emergency work, such as difficult airway, anaphylaxis, and invasive procedures.

As ambulatory surgery becomes more extensive, it will also be necessary to make the ambulatory unit an area of education and training for medical students, surgeons, anesthesiologists, and nurses. This should be recognized as requiring dedicated resources, such as instructors, and potentially delaying case performance and turnover while remaining compatible with high-quality care provision and effective running [11]. A model for surgical education is to have a senior surgeon ready to take over if a case is prolonged beyond certain limits, or having the trainee do the case with the senior surgeon supervising.

References

1. Toftgaard C, Parmentier G. International terminology in ambulatory surgery and its worldwide practice. In: Lemos P, Jarrett P, Philip B, eds. *Day Surgery – Development and Practice*, London: IAAS, 2006: 35–60.

2. Jarrett P, Staniszewski A. The development of ambulatory surgery and future challenges. In: Lemos P, Jarrett P, Philip B, eds. *Day Surgery – Development and Practice*, London: IAAS, 2006: 21–34.

3. Warner MA, Shields SE, Chute CG. Major morbidity and mortality within 1 month of ambulatory surgery and anesthesia. *JAMA* 1993;270:1437–41.

4. Engbaek J, Bartholdy J, Hjortso NC. Return hospital visits and morbidity within 60 days after day surgery: a retrospective study of 18,736 day surgical procedures. *Acta Anaesthesiol Scand* 2006;50:911–19.

5. Vila H, Jr., Soto R, Cantor AB, Mackey D. Comparative outcomes analysis of procedures performed in physician offices and ambulatory surgery centers. *Arch Surg* 2003;138:991–5.

6. Grogaard B, Kimsas E, Raeder J. Wound infection in day-surgery. *Ambul Surg* 2001;9:109–12.

7. Holtz TH, Wenzel RP. Postdischarge surveillance for nosocomial wound infection: a brief review and commentary. *Am J Infect Control* 1992;20:206–13.

8. Rasmussen LS. Postoperative cognitive dysfunction: incidence and prevention. *Best Pract Res Clin Anaesthesiol* 2006;20:315–30.

9. Canet J, Raeder J, Rasmussen LS, et al. Cognitive dysfunction after minor surgery in the elderly. *Acta Anaesthesiol Scand* 2003;47:1204–10.

10. Ward B, Imarengiaye C, Peirovy J, Chung F. Cognitive function is minimally impaired after ambulatory surgery. *Can J Anaesth* 2005;52:1017–21.

11. Skattum J, Edwin B, Trondsen E, et al. Outpatient laparoscopic surgery: feasibility and consequences for education and health care costs. *Surg Endosc* 2004;18:796–801.

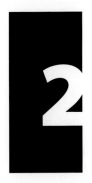

2 Organization of ambulatory surgery and anesthesia

Physical organization [1]

There are different levels of organizing ambulatory surgery; everything from a single ambulatory case performed between scheduled inpatient procedures in an inpatient organization to freestanding, complete hospitals dedicated completely to ambulatory care.

The single ambulatory patient integrated in an inpatient organization

This implies that occasional inpatients are treated as ambulatory; that is, they are discharged in the afternoon or evening after surgery instead of staying overnight. This is assessed individually for each case and patient, and may be planned in advance or organized ad hoc as a consequence of uneventful surgery and recovery, or perhaps as a request from the patient or personnel, "Is there any reason for this patient to stay in the hospital overnight?"

It is hard to see much advantage of the ambulatory approach when it is applied in this way. The hospital cannot plan to employ fewer staff (thus making savings) during evenings and overnight and the patient is exposed to the full hospital experience with its potential for delays, cumbersome case flow, and less consistent exchange of information. However, it may be beneficial for the patient to go home even if an overnight stay had been planned or is the rule, provided that analgesia, anti-emesis, and safety are well taken care of. This model may be the only option in units where the majority of patients are inpatients, or in very small hospitals that, as a rule, only provide inpatient care.

This may also be a model when trying to expand ambulatory care to new patient categories. In such a situation ambulatory care may be introduced very gently by saying to everyone (patient, surgeon, staff) in advance:

> Mr./Mrs. X is an inpatient and planned to be treated as an inpatient; we will go through the full inpatient routine and have an overnight bed ready. However, when surgery is finished and if the recovery and total situation are uneventful, we will evaluate the case for basic discharge criteria. If these are all fulfilled we will send the patient home.

Thus, the model may work as a pilot project for expanding day care. The next step may be to say, "We have two similar patients, both planned as inpatients, but we expect that at least one of them will go home, thus we will only plan for one overnight bed."

Then the project may be expanded to three or four patients and when it becomes evident that most of these patients actually go home, you have effectively established a new ambulatory patient treatment chain very smoothly, and may then move to the next phase of saying, "These will be ambulatory cases, but we still need options available for inpatient care in some cases, either planned or unplanned."

The ambulatory program as part of an inpatient program or organization

This means that you deliberately plan for an ambulatory program as a minor part of the ordinary inpatient setting. It may be necessary to dedicate a specific day and/or operating theater to ambulatory care, or, more commonly, to plan one or more weekdays where at least one theater is reserved for ambulatory care. Once the ambulatory care becomes a planned issue for a defined number of patients or category of patients, you may be in a position to dedicate the following to the ambulatory setting both preoperatively and postoperatively: instructions, methods of communication, consultant surgeons' time, and postoperative care, i.e., minimizing opioids, minimizing nausea, encourage mobilization, etc. While there may be dedicated personnel for the ambulatory cases or days, they will probably have to participate as inpatient workers rather than being full-time and working fully trained in the ambulatory setting. A pragmatic solution is to have some secretaries, preoperative nurses, and postoperative nurses fully dedicated to the ambulatory patients on those days when the ambulatory program is followed. Also the surgeons and anesthesiologists should sign up to the philosophy of the ambulatory program in terms of their attitudes toward information exchange and focusing on uneventful and fast recovery. Despite this, patients may still experience much of the cumbersome inpatient routines, and the hospital may not be in a position to make financial savings as the limited and often unpredictable number of ambulatory patients within the dominantly inpatient setting may be hard to translate into real changes in organization, staffing, and thus economy. Still this model may be a good alternative in small hospitals with so few ambulatory cases that they cannot justify having a separate unit running five full days a week.

The ambulatory unit integrated into an inpatient hospital

This occurs when there are enough ambulatory patients to run an ambulatory unit, but major facilities must be provided by the inpatient hospital. The unit runs five full days a week, but there may also be a unit staffed by part-time workers on either short days or short weeks. In order to be called a separate unit (different from the model in Section 2.1.2) there should be an area and personnel dedicated fully to ambulatory care. Usually this is a unit with at least a reception area and a phase II recovery and discharge area. Often it will also include preoperative holding and phase I recovery areas (i.e., the postoperative care unit, PACU). The integration with inpatients usually occurs in the operating theater, which is part of the inpatient hospital facility, but with specific days or theaters dedicated to ambulatory care.

The benefit of this organization is that it enables the hospital to take full advantage of employing a dedicated ambulatory staff for all preoperative and postoperative care, and of providing the patient with the comfort of not being exposed to the full hospital setting. The hospital may attain better cost-efficiency through the shared use of expensive theaters and specialized equipment for an increased total number of hours per week than can be achieved with two fully separate locations. The downside remains the demanding logistics implicit in coordinating those parts of the treatment pathways that are shared with inpatients. Problems may arise through having personnel who are not dedicated to ambulatory care and the potential for cancellation of the ambulatory program should the inpatient organization become overloaded with emergency cases.

The freestanding ambulatory unit inside the inpatient hospital

This occurs when the ambulatory program is run totally separately from inpatient program; including having its own premises, and dedicated pre-, per-, and postoperative staff, with the exception of maybe the surgeons and anesthesiologists, who are often employed by the "mother" hospital. The doctors may be available for ambulatory care on a case-by-case basis, for a full list or a full day, for a limited period, or as a permanent employee. The good aspect of this model is that a sophisticated hospital providing backup for extra testing and unexpected emergencies is close by and easily accessible. An unexpected transition to inpatient care or the need for prolonged recovery is usually easily achieved. There will also be the potential for some flexibility in the use of very expensive equipment and flexibility on the part of the doctors, who may manage their time across in-hospital tasks and ambulatory care. This has good and bad aspects: a flexible day may mean that an ambulatory case has to wait for a doctor who is not dedicated to the ambulatory program and busy with something else in another part of the hospital. Experience shows that with all models of ambulatory care that are provided close to the rest of the hospital, the nurses will spend some time and effort bleeping the doctors, who are working constantly across the site.

Having fully separated units makes it easier to account for cost-efficiency measures, and to have separate budgets and accounting. It also makes it easier to promote team-working and to enable everyone in the treatment chain to reap the benefits of efficient working. This acts as an incentive to get the lists done without delay so as to avoid having to remain after hours as no one from the inpatient hospital is available to take over these duties in the evening or overnight.

The freestanding ambulatory unit as a satellite of the inpatient hospital

This is a model in which the ambulatory unit is physically separate from the rest of the hospital, either at the end of a long corridor or in a separate building some distance away. The idea is to be far enough away from the rest of the hospital that doctors and other personnel will be unable to leave the unit between cases, while being close enough for any extra tests, access to expertise, or unplanned admissions to be achieved fairly easy. Making the doctors stay in the unit usually eliminates the problem of their not being available to start the next case, and it usually also speeds up other parts of the treatment, as doctors are more likely to use any small break to talk with the patients, finish patient reports, and be more involved in the ambulatory team. Being geographically distant also protects the ambulatory personnel from being moved to provide inpatient care if the main hospital is experiencing staff shortages, is overworked and understaffed, or there are other problems in running the inpatient unit. The downsides of being at a distance are the somewhat more demanding logistics for patient transportation when extra tests or evaluations are needed or in cases of an unplanned admission.

The freestanding ambulatory unit or hospital

Freestanding hospital

This has all the benefits of being a separate unit in terms of personnel, routines, and economy. The downside may be the need to bring in extra services which have to be organized and usually paid for. If the ambulatory hospital is big enough, many of these extra services may be part of the organization, such as laboratories, cardiology services, radiology services and so on, and they may even be set up to arrange unplanned overnight stays if needed. There will always be some need for the patient with a rare and serious complication to be admitted to an inpatient hospital, and this should be included in the planning. For smaller freestanding units there may be two ways of obtaining external service. The first is to have established connections and systems for making appointments with a neighboring inpatient hospital; the alternative is to limit the need for such services as much as possible. The latter may be accomplished by having a narrow selection of procedures on offer and then to focus on optimizing the selective "production line" within the organization. Further one can try to avoid trouble by only taking healthy patients assessed as grade I or II according to the American Society of Anesthesiologists (ASA) status, with a well-organized family situation, who live close by, and so on.

Freestanding office based

These units almost always concentrate on a narrow selection of procedures, for instance doing solely ear, nose and throat (ENT), solely plastic surgery, solely dental surgery, and so on. Most of them will also place restraints on the patient's general health and social situation, in order to avoid serious complications and problems. These units may be very efficient because they can make very stable and tight teams with logistics focused solely on one type of patient and surgery. They may be more pragmatic and less dogmatic than larger clinics in terms of what personnel and routines are actually needed; for instance, not having excess scrub staff and drapes, not having fully certified nurses as assistants, and so on. Problems for such units are then ensuring that they fulfill all the requirements for safe running and that they have proper backup routines for any potentially dangerous events. They may be lulled into a false sense of security because they have a fairly low number of cases compared with a big hospital and as a consequence have infrequent exposure to problems. Then, should a very rare and occasionally serious complication happen, the whole clinic may be under threat and investigated to see whether their formal safety aspects and backup routines were adequate.

What is the optimal size of a unit?

Unit size is usually defined as the number of theaters and surgical teams working simultaneously within it. Two major trends are important in this context: (1) the bigger the unit's size the greater its potential for synergy effects of logistics, personnel, and equipment serving more than one team at a time; (2) the bigger the unit's size the greater the amount of effort needed to organize, coordinate, and plan the work it carries out. Bigger units are more flexible in some ways, for example in their ability to handle staff sick leave smoothly, and to manage the unpredictable length of some cases, cancellations, and any extra services required unexpectedly.

Having only one theater may work well and efficiently if the turnover time between patients is not too great. This means that minimal time should be spent on cleaning and draping and that there should be enough instruments to allow for smooth running, avoiding delays while equipment is sterilized.

With two theaters, two full teams may work in parallel or, if the cases are numerous and short, one surgeon may go between the theaters, which optimizes the efficient use of their time. In systems with nurse-anesthetists, synergy may be achieved by having one anesthesiologist serving two theaters concomitantly, with one nurse in each. With three theaters and a nurse-anesthetist in each, even more efficient use of the anesthesiologist may be possible when the cases are straightforward. However, when increasing the unit size to more than three or four theaters, some of the synergistic effects on secretarial help, the anesthesiologist, and supporting functions may be challenged. When an organization grows there is synergy up to a certain size over which there is a need to employ more people such that much of the synergy and savings may be lost unless one expands a little further. With more than two to three theaters in a unit, it may also be practical sometimes to split a big unit into two separately run organizations within the same geographical premises.

What is needed for safe practice? [2]

Safety will be regulated by laws and standards in most countries. There may be separate standards for unit accreditation, for personnel qualification, and for safe way of practicing. In Norway this has been put together into a national standard for safe anesthetic practice, which focuses on personnel qualification and attendance, equipment for monitoring and emergencies, as well as on the physical premises. With this approach there is no formal need for accreditation, but units are obliged to adhere to the standard and can be accused of malpractice if they do not and something goes wrong [2]. Much of what is stated below comes from this standard, and most of it will be common with standards in other countries and with common sense.

A major basic rule is to have the same level of standards, safety, and quality for ambulatory care as for inpatient surgery.

The physical requirement

There is a need for separate areas for preoperative care, the operation, and for postoperative care. In an office-based setting these may all be in the same office if the surgery is minor or contaminated (i.e., ENT, proctology, vaginal gynecology). Otherwise, the demands of minimal contamination will require a separate operating theater with increased standards for washing, draping, and hygiene of the personnel. In the operating theater there should be a dedicated telephone or calling system or emergency button for immediately summoning assistance in critical situations. In office-based settings it is especially important to pay attention to facilities for resuscitation, access to the trolley, and enabling the transportation of the patient on a stretcher out of the unit and into an ambulance. Also elevator breakdown should be considered, with either access to a stairway that is large enough for a stretcher to pass or a setup with a semi-upright stretcher that may be easier to take down a narrow stairway.

The preoperative area may be divided into a reception area (in which the patient wears their daily clothes), a holding area (in which they are dressed in a hospital gown and ready for surgery), and in some cases an induction room for anesthesia or establishment of blocks. The postoperative area may be divided into a PACU with monitoring of the patient's vital functions and a phase II recovery area with no technical monitoring in which the patient sits in a chair waiting for discharge. Furthermore there should be a room for private conversations and consultation with patients individually. In units with a mixture of children and adults it is wise to have a separate area for the children, and even further separation for children who are crying and distressed. Separate areas for children are also mandated because of the need to involve parents more extensively in all phases of the stay, except the operation itself.

The pre- and postoperative areas may be completely different (pull-through organization – patient comes into the hospital via one route and leaves via a different one) or the same (the patient leaves one area for surgery and returns to it afterwards, called race-track organization – patient comes into and leaves the hospital via the same route). The benefits of a race-track organization are that the patients are treated by the same nursing staff before and after surgery, the postoperative premises are familiar, and the staff are better employed throughout the day, with predominantly preoperative care early on and postoperative care at the end of the day. The benefits of a pull-through organization are that preoperative patients do not intermingle with postoperative patients and relatives, the premises and personnel can be more fully dedicated to either pre- or postoperative (e.g., monitoring, resting chairs) care, and it is easier to keep good track of where patients are in the perioperative process. Generally, a race-track organization is best for small units (or big units if they are subdivided) whereas a pull-through organization is best for big units.

Equipment

Basic perioperative monitoring equipment should be ready: noninvasive blood pressure monitoring, electrocardiography (ECG), pulse oximetry, capnography for all intubations, gas monitoring (both in and out of patients) of oxygen and all inhalational gases, alarms to alert to problems of gas delivery and a low oxygen content in the ventilation gas, and temperature monitoring. In units carrying out more extensive surgery and/or for elderly, fragile patients the ability to measure blood pressure invasively should be an option. However, a pulse oximeter may be the only monitoring needed for healthy patients having limited surgery. Spare oxygen bottles should always be ready for immediate use, and scavenger systems should be present for all inhalational anesthetics.

In case of emergencies there must be fast access to a suction device, a self-expanding ventilation bag with reservoir and extra oxygen supply, a defibrillator and emergency drugs, and an intubation kit including devices for difficult intubations (i.e., stylet, laryngeal mask, extra laryngoscope, emergency tracheotomy kit, and preferably some sort of fiberoptic or visualizing intubation device).

The postoperative care unit should be equipped for routine monitoring of blood pressure, ECG, and pulse oximetry, as well as with a full emergency backup kit as described above.

Personnel

The need for various personnel and their qualifications will vary between countries due to different traditions in training and standards. The access to nurse-anesthetists may vary considerably between different countries as will also their qualifications and daily tasks.

In general there should always be an anesthesiologist responsible for the unit's setup, routines, and also for accepting and planning individual patients for anesthesia.

a. **General anesthesia:** a basic setup is to have a qualified anesthesiologist doing the case alone, from preoperative evaluation, through induction of anesthesia, to postoperative care. Although alone, the anesthetist will usually have an assistant or technicians with him or her, and one of the scrub nurses may also be prepared to help in the event of unexpected problems. In many countries a nurse-anesthetist will maintain the anesthetic assisted by the doctor during induction and emergence, and in most countries nurses will take care of postoperative surveillance with the doctor there as a backup. In some countries it is a requirement to have a trained assistant (who may be a nurse-anesthetist) always working together with the anesthesiologist for general anesthesia.

b. **Sedation** (see also Sedation): anesthesiological training and qualification should be mandatory for all cases of deep sedation, that is any case where there is a risk of obstructed airway or apnea. Recently European guidelines have been established for this kind of practice, stating that a dedicated and specifically trained person (i.e., nurse, nurse-anesthetist, or doctor) should be in charge of anything other than awake sedation, being dedicated to that task and the individual patient continuously [3]. Awake sedation with moderate doses of approved conventional opioids (i.e., morphine, meperidine, oxycodone, etc.) or benzodiazepines is allowed to be given by any doctor, who is ultimately responsible for that treatment. The use of a pulse oximeter is required as is the dedicated and continuous surveillance of the patient.

c. **Local anesthesia**: may be used by doctors in general, but care should be taken to obey the rules of maximum dosing and toxicity, especially important in plastic surgery where large doses sometimes are used and fatalities have occurred.

d. **Regional anesthesia**: regional anesthesia should generally be reserved for trained anesthesiologists, although some surgeons are adequately trained in dedicated blocks for eye surgery and hernia surgery as well as in intravenous regional anesthesia. As to spinal or epidural anesthesia, these blocks should only be done by anesthesiologists and monitored by anesthesia-trained personnel. Qualified, continual anesthetic monitoring is mandatory throughout these cases in order to respond to the cardiovascular status of the patient.

e. **Postoperative care unit**: in the PACU the patients should be watched by nurses specially trained in monitoring and the handling of emergencies of ventilation, circulation, and surgical complications (i.e., bleeding). They are also required to have appropriate knowledge of pain and nausea evaluation and treatment. A dedicated person should watch the patient continuously as long as they are unconscious, and immediate access to anesthesiologists or an intensivist should be possible.

Documentation
Basic documentation

All units should have a regularly updated collection of documents (paper and/or electronic) relevant to their practice. ISO (International Organization for Standardization) certification may be a way to establish all routines optimally, but most of the components and standards of ISO certification should be present in all units anyway:

- User manual for all *equipment*, service routines, spare parts, and backup systems in the case of failure
- Routines for *personnel*: how to recruit, ensure proper standards, education and continuous training, emergency drills, clear-cut definitions of responsibilities, and reporting of problems
- Routines for *running* the unit and individual cases: what is needed in terms of equipment, drugs and personnel, patients' and procedural requirements, detailed charts of patient flow, clear-cut routines for PACU discharge, unit discharge, pre- and postoperative follow-up, routines for different potential medical emergencies, etc.

Individual documentation of each case

There should be an anesthetic report for each patient, as with inpatients. The report may be manual (easily readable!) or electronic or mixed. A list of contents will include:

- Patient identification
- Date and time notations for patient flow and all drugs given
- Preoperative diagnoses, preoperative health, ASA class
- Equipment in use and signed preoperative check
- Patient position and type of surgery
- All drugs given and code for type of anesthesia
- Vital signs, ventilator setting, and intravenous (iv) pump rates every fifth minute
- Documentation of all problems and their handling
- Names of all personnel involved and the names of the responsible anesthesiologist and surgeon
- Postoperative orders
- Documentation on report (time and patient's status) given to postoperative personnel.

In the *postoperative phase*:

- Regular documentation on vital signs as long as the patient is unconscious
- Documentation (time and criteria) for PACU discharge readiness, PACU discharge, and unit discharge
- Documentation of all drugs given and all information given, especially about important potential complications and how to get immediate and adequate contact with health care services on a 24-h basis
- A copy of the *written report from the surgeon* should follow the patient at discharge and also be available to any health care facilities where the patient may call during the hours and days after discharge in the case of an emergency
- After discharge there should be a *quality control system* (letter, phone, visit) for all or selected patients and a system for being notified about all serious problems or unanticipated admissions (see Chapter 7).

References

1. Jarrett P, Roberts L. Planning and designing a day surgery unit. In: Lemos P, Jarrett P, Philip B, eds. *Day Surgery – Development and Practice*, London: IAAS, 2006: 61–88.

2. Gisvold SE, Raeder J, Jyssum T, et al. Guidelines for the practice of anesthesia in Norway. *Acta Anaesthesiol Scand* 2002;46:942–6.

3. Knape JT, Adriaensen H, van Aken H, et al. Guidelines for sedation and/or analgesia by non-anaesthesiology doctors. *Eur J Anaesthesiol* 2007;24:563–7.

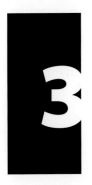

Procedure and patient selection, pre-admittance preparation

Procedure selection: which procedures are not suited for ambulatory surgery

Procedures for which extensive pretreatment is needed

For some elective procedures specialized pretreatment in the hospital will be needed, e.g., extensive gastrointestinal lavage, intravenous drug therapy, or radiologic marking of structures. If, for these reasons, the patient has to stay in hospital the night before the operation, the case will not fall within the definition of ambulatory care, even though same-day discharge may be possible.

Procedures for which the postoperative condition is incompatible with same-day discharge

Suitability for the vast majority of procedures for ambulatory care will depend on the patient's condition within the first few hours after the procedure, which depends on a combination of the patient's general health and characteristics of the surgical procedure and anesthetic technique. The bottom line is whether you expect the patient to fulfill the discharge criteria (see Appendix 3.1) by the end of the day at the unit.

If, for any reason, qualified medical observation or treatment beyond the first few hours after the end of surgery or after the ambulatory unit closes is likely, the patient should be planned as an inpatient. This is likely to be the case for most kinds of *emergency surgery*; in such cases the preoperative preparation may be incomplete, the diagnoses may be unclear, the patient may be in an unstable physiologic condition, and there will most often be a need for treatment and medical observation afterwards.

Similarly, in some elective patients their general health condition and/or the nature of their surgical procedure implies postoperative instability with a need for close medical follow-up. Inpatient status is usually necessary for most major procedures on an open abdomen, thorax, or skull for reasons of major blood loss or fluid shifts, strong postoperative pain, postoperative need for intravenous fluids or specialized substrates, or specialized care of postoperative wounds or drains. Further, procedures leaving the patient unable to mobilize, not fully awake, or unable to consume oral fluids or tablets within the deadline for discharge will not be suitable for ambulatory care.

Discharge criteria

When planning for ambulatory care it is important and useful to have a specified list of discharge criteria (see Table 6.5, page 149) in mind. If you suspect that the patient in question will probably not fulfill all items on the list on the afternoon or evening of the day of the

Table 3.1. Examples of advanced procedures successfully carried out in an ambulatory setting

- Laparoscopic major gastric surgery [2,3]:
  - cholecystectomy, fundoplication, gastric banding (obese)
- Laparoscopic major gynecology:
  - hysterectomy [4]
- Mini-invasive low-back surgery [5]
- Breast cancer surgery [6]
- Bladder/prostate [7] cancer surgery
- Cruciate ligament repair [8]
- Open shoulder surgery [9]
- Major plastic surgery [10]
  - breast reduction, abdominal fat reduction
- Thyroidectomy [11]
- Tonsillectomy [12]

operation, the procedure should not be done ambulatory. Within this scope it is also necessary to evaluate complications that may arise during home travel or home stay, based on the nature of the patient's surgery and anesthetic. This should be weighed against the ease of getting to the nearest suitable health care provider. The important issue is to decide whether a "*a worst case scenario*" for the individual case could be handled safely under ambulatory care. If the worst case scenario is strong pain (e.g., orthopedic limb surgery), this may be very well treated by an able doctor far away from any hospital. However, if the worst case is gastrointestinal leakage into the peritoneum, or deep infection (e.g., laparoscopies), it may be appropriate to have the patient within a few hours' reach of a surgical hospital. When there is a danger of severe bleeding (e.g., tonsillectomy), the patient should never be more than 30–60 minutes away from a hospital that can provide adequate ENT service for controlling the bleed as well as transfusion, emergency surgery and anesthetic care if needed.

In these circumstances the use of an ordinary hotel or patient hotel near to the hospital may facilitate the use of ambulatory care even for patients living at very remote locations.

The types of procedure that can be done in an ambulatory setting are growing and Table 3.1 gives examples of some fairly extensive procedures reported as having been achieved successfully.

Patient selection: which patients are not suited for ambulatory care? [1]

This section discusses patient selection from the standpoint of having a patient booked in for a potentially ambulatory surgical procedure. The particular preparations and precautions to enable ambulatory care, if deemed appropriate, are discussed. The handling of the patient on the day of surgery is discussed further in Chapter 5.

General considerations

All patients should be sent back to their home environment on the day of surgery *unless* their own health status combined with the surgery and anesthetic indicate that a stay in hospital is required to ensure adequate safety and quality of care. Again, it is important to assess the discharge criteria and ascertain whether they are likely to be fulfilled (see above).

A general rule is that the patient should *consent* to being sent home; that is, the patient should feel safe and ready to cooperate on the measures and precautions that need to be taken after discharge. Further, the patient should arrange for a responsible chaperone to be with them until the next day. This also includes patients who are discharged to hotels or hospital-hotels; someone should be in the room (or suite) until the next day, unless there is a more extensive patient hotel setting with regular or automatic monitoring of a patient's vital functions in the room.

The *length of travel home* is not decisive per se, rather the important issues are whether a "worst case scenario" during the journey home can be adequately handled (see above) or whether the patient is motivated for the journey in question.

In patients with drug, alcohol, or substance abuse or who have an unstable social situation, there should be a low threshold for planning for inpatient status, again based on an individual evaluation of quality and safety with a "worst case scenario" in mind.

Ideally the evaluation to select between inpatient and outpatient care should be done shortly before planned surgery. This ensures relevance on the day of surgery with minimal chance of cancellation, but should be far enough in advance to allow for extra tests to be taken, specialist consultations to be made, and good planning of the operating list to be undertaken.

Some days in advance may be the minimum for having these options and 1–3 weeks may be optimal, whereas making the evaluation a long time in advance may increase the risk of the patient's condition changing from that stated and planned for during the preoperative evaluation. Despite this, a full history, physical examination, and test results obtained within 3–6 months before the actual day of surgery may be acceptable for scheduling a day of surgery. If more than 3–6 months has elapsed, then most units will require a new visit for preoperative planning, or at least that a physician calls the patient to ask about any changes in condition.

In many places there is a separate anesthesiological consult prior to all ambulatory surgery, either in conjunction with the patient's visit to the surgeon or as a separate visit some days or weeks ahead of the planned surgery. The pattern of these visits may also be influenced by the financial setup or billing system; if a reasonable fee is involved, the tendency is for all patients to visit. If the patient is not especially ill and the anesthesiologist insists on the patient making a separate visit to him/her, this is not good total economy. Also it may be a waste of the anesthesiologist's time to see all patients in the preoperative surgical consultation period.

My experience is that surgeons talk with their patients, and are able to identify those ASA I and II patients whom they do not need to see before the day of surgery unless the patient makes a specific request. The surgeon or the nurse will make a checklist of the patient's health (compiled from patient self-evaluation), which will be seen by the anesthesiologist the day before surgery. If the patient has ASA III or IV status, the surgeon will either send them for anesthesiological consultation before surgery, or make a telephone consultation with the anesthesiologist while the patient is in their office. This may be the most efficient way forward as a quick telephone can sort out: whether the patient is OK for scheduling, whether the surgeon should order any tests or an internist consult, whether special information about drugs should be given, or whether the patient should have a consult with the anesthesiologist.

It will always remain the responsibility of the surgeon and anesthesiologist in charge of the case on the day of surgery to ensure that the indication is still valid and that no major change in general health has occurred. If there is a change in situation this will always require an individual evaluation of what to do, namely to go ahead as planned, to postpone the case to later in the day (to allow time for extra tests or consult), to postpone to another day, or to cancel.

Patient health

Everyone who admits patients to ambulatory surgical treatment and an anesthetic should know the ASA classification (Appendix 3.1).

All ASA I and II patients should be considered healthy enough to receive ambulatory care. This includes uncomplicated (i.e., no accompanying disorders) patients with obesity and elderly patients. ASA III and ASA IV patients should be evaluated individually for their suitability for ambulatory care. Serious health problems, psychiatric disorders, and mental/cognitive deficits are not necessarily contraindications, and stable ASA III and sometimes even ASA IV patients may be treated in an ambulatory setting [13]. The important issue is whether the patient's condition is considered to be stable and under control, and furthermore that the added stress of surgery plus anesthetic will not render the patient unsuitable for an ambulatory setup.

Special patient conditions: impact on selection, planning, and applied care

Patient selection will also be influenced by the type of unit, especially the readiness of access to expert help and equipment during a case if needed, and the logistics of unplanned admission. If the ambulatory unit is within a large multipurpose hospital, it may even be planned with an ambulatory setup for patients with a 50:50 chance of requiring inpatient care, because overnight wards are present in the same building or hospital. In a downtown freestanding unit with a longer journey time to hospital such a 50:50 case should not generally be planned for outpatient care.

Patient age

Children [14,15]

The newborn infant -- Newborn patients require special equipment and competence for anesthesia and surgical treatment whether as an inpatient or in the ambulatory setting; the question is whether sending the infant home will be safe. The main concerns include major fluid shifts, poor tolerance of problems with oral hydration and nutrition, and problems relating to respiratory control and airway maintenance. The social and parental situation should also be taken into consideration: are the parents able to interpret signs of problems? Also, will they understand when they need to contact the hospital for a consultation? Will the setting after discharge be compatible with handling a "worst case scenario?"

While term-born infants are probably at no extra risk from same-day discharge, concerns over airway and airway control remain, especially when opioids have been used or the child has been intubated. For these reasons, most units do not accept children less than 3–6 months old for ambulatory surgery, except for minor superficial procedures carried out with local anesthesia. Further, if there is any doubt about the safety aspects or the infant has respiratory problems during recovery, they should generally be kept in hospital overnight.

The newborn ex-premature infant -- Prematurely born infants have a disturbance of breathing control, which may develop into apnea during the first day after general anesthesia, intravenous sedation or opioid use. Much debate has taken place about what is a safe age limit for same-day discharge in these patients, and some extra risk seems to be present until at least 50–55 weeks post-conception. This means that these patients should be treated as inpatients for surgery done within 3–4 months of their planned full-term date. Again, if severely premature or there is any doubt, it is wise to extend the inpatient rule for at least a further 1–2 months.

Children in general –– Children above the age of 3–6 months are generally excellent candidates for the ambulatory setting for many reasons: they are usually otherwise fairly healthy, they definitely feel happier at home than in hospital, and the surgery is usually well suited to the ambulatory setting, being superficial, short lasting, and well suited for local anesthesia as an adjuvant per- and postoperatively. Also children with severe cognitive impairment or psychiatric disease usually benefit from remaining in the hospital environment for as short a time as possible, with a rapid, same-day return to their normal environment and carers [16]. The general rules for ambulatory patient and surgery selection also apply to children.

The child with sleep apnea syndrome –– Children with clear symptoms of sleep apnea syndrome (SAS; see later) should be admitted overnight after general anesthesia or any technique involving perioperative opioid. Usually SAS in children is caused by being over-weight or having big tonsils. Despite removing the tonsils (i.e., tonsillectomy) there may be an ongoing risk of SAS during the first postoperative night because peritonsillar tissue needs a day to adapt after surgery. As most tonsillectomy patients younger than 3 years have SAS, the general rule is not to send these patients home on the same day as surgery.

The child with a runny nose –– The general rule is to wait for 1–2 weeks after a common cold or upper airway infection, however this may be hard to achieve in children with frequent airway problems. A history should be taken to document the child's present level of activity, eating, playing with friends, presence of fever, and so on. If the child is in his/her usual normal functioning state with a concomitant runny nose, surgery and anesthesia may proceed. If the child is worse than usual, shows any sign of bacterial or lower airway infection, fever, or fatigue, or is not playing or eating as usual, the case should be postponed. Where there is doubt it may help to auscultate the lung sounds and take the rectal temperature and a blood sample to check for normal C-reactive protein (CRP) and leukocyte levels before proceeding. A runny nose may be a further indication not to intubate, unless it is unavoidable.

The child with asthma or episodes of laryngitis (pseudocroup) –– Children with asthma or episodes of laryngitis should, if possible, have their surgery during those periods of few attacks, and always receive optimal pretreatment with their usual drugs and aerosols. Intubation should only be carried out upon a strong indication, and then special care should be taken to avoid using an endotracheal tube that has a tight fit within the trachea. Maintenance with inhalational agents may lower airway irritability, and ketamine may be considered if wheezing occurs perioperatively and is not resolved by sevoflurane or isoflurane administration. If the child has a wheeze preoperatively the case should usually be postponed; however, if wheezing is always present, the case should probably be scheduled as an inpatient.

Old age, elderly

An elderly patient with cognitive impairment may very well have ambulatory surgery, provided they normally have adequate function at their place of residence (home or institution).

As with children, they will profit from being away from their familiar environment for as short a time as possible. It has been shown [17] that elderly patients having a hernia repair are significantly less likely to have cognitive dysfunction 1 week after ambulatory treatment compared with 1 week after inpatient care. There was also an insignificant tendency in favor of ambulatory care after 3 months, but the 1-year follow-up data were similar to those of the general age-matched population. Although one should bear in mind that even the very healthy elderly patient has limited physiological reserves (lungs, heart, kidneys, etc.) compared with a younger cohort, the evaluation of whether ambulatory care is appropriate should be based on their concomitant disease, the type of surgery, and their psychosocial situation, as with other patients. It is important to obtain the baseline blood pressure in elderly patients, as they often have increased stiffness of the cardiovascular system and raised systolic blood pressure. Also, a 12-lead ECG should be taken routinely for all elderly patients above the age of 65. If the planned procedure is only a superficial one being carried out with local anesthesia without deep sedation, the ECG may be omitted if the patient has a negative history, because important aspects of the ECG will be display routinely via on the one-lead perioperative monitoring. The one-lead ECG is displayed before any drugs are given and will provide information about arrhythmia, P-Q prolongation, or heart block and any ST segment changes in the precordial area. The one-lead ECG cannot provide information about signs of heart failure, hypertrophy and previous infarction; however, these factors will not significantly influence your handling of a minor case in patients with a negative history.

Patients with airway or pulmonary disease

Breathing disorders may be classified as problems with airways and lungs, with respiratory control, or with the muscular function of breathing.

Patients with an episode of infection should generally be postponed until 1–2 weeks after the infection has fully resolved. The exception may be the child with a constant runny nose (see above). Also adults with very mild or declining symptoms of upper airway viral infection, not affecting their general daily function, who are presenting for minor or intermediately invasive procedures may be accepted. If a postoperative sore throat or coughing is likely to be a problem in light of the surgical procedure, such as with hernia repair and surgery in the neck or breast area, mild viral symptoms indicate that the case should be postponed.

Smokers should be strongly advised not to smoke on the day of surgery, as a small amount of carbon monoxide reduces hemoglobin's oxygen-binding capacity for hours. There is usually no need to cancel the case if the patient has smoked preoperatively. However, having surgery is a good opportunity to try to convince patients to stop smoking. Ideally they should stop at least 3–4 weeks ahead of surgery, because airway irritability and secretion production often reactively increase in the first few weeks after smoking cessation.

For patients with severe airway or pulmonary disease or infections, a more thorough approach should be undertaken for preoperative evaluation. The patient's history should be taken, to include: ability to walk two flights of stairs, the amount of coughing and secretions, as well as episodic changes versus stability of their condition. Preoperative lung radiographs, arterial blood gas, and spirometry with vital capacity and forced expiratory volume in one second (FEV_1), with and without bronchodilator, are further options. Generally, a vital capacity of less than 1.5–2 liters in an adult or an FEV_1 of less than 1–1.5 liters indicates an increased likelihood of needing ventilatory support and inpatient status postoperatively.

Even so, patients who have severe pulmonary disease but who have stable function in their daily environment should still be considered for ambulatory care provided the planned procedure is compatible with the situation at home to which they would return afterwards. However, a low threshold should be anticipated for transferring such ambulatory cases to an inpatient status upon evaluation postoperatively.

Sleep apnea syndrome (SAS)

Sleep apnea syndrome is underdiagnosed, but probably occurs in 4% of the adult male population and in 2% of females. It is associated with obesity and also with large tonsils or adenoids, especially in small children, but can be present without any of these [18]. Although these patients manage at home preoperatively, their chances of respiratory arrest are increased in particular during the first night after surgery with general anesthesia or following the administration of postoperative opioids. Although fatalities are very rare, eight cases were reported in a large American survey [19] and one case is one too many and could be avoided by being an inpatient overnight with continuous monitoring.

The symptoms of SAS almost always include snoring but should be accompanied by more problems to be confident of the diagnosis: respiratory arrest (>10 s), frequent change in position while asleep, being tired in spite of a normal "length of sleep," morning headache, and a family history of SAS. A more specific and detailed diagnosis can be made with polysomnography, in which the patient is monitored continuously for a full night with pulse oximetry and ECG, and the number and lengths of apnea episodes are recorded. More than 30 episodes of hypopnea or apnea per hour signals a serious condition whereas fewer than 15 is mild. The fairly precise prediction of a serious condition can be made clinically if the patient tests positively on these four anamnestic items: loud snoring (heard through a wall or door), observed apnea during sleep, being tired in spite of normal length of sleep in bed, and hypertension [20].

A rational approach to these patients is shown in Table 3.2.

Importantly, when these patients are planned for inpatient care, an ordinary stay on the ward will not be adequate; they must be monitored continuously during the night. A pulse oximeter may suffice, although signs of hypoxia are somewhat delayed so the optimal situation is to link the patient to a respiratory rate monitor with apnea alarm.

Table 3.2. Rational approach to assessing patients with SAS

Known SAS	If treated with CPAP → OK as ambulatory[a] If loco-regional and no opioids postoperatively → OK If seriously affected/general anesthesia/opioids → inpatient with monitoring!
Suspected SAS	If serious symptoms → polysomnography (or treat as inpatient) Mild symptoms (not tired, no major apnea or distress) → OK if no opioid effects after discharge
Otherwise	Morbidly obese, no SAS mentioned: ask for symptoms, obtain partner/parent information. If in doubt → plan as inpatient

[a] It has been shown that SAS patients who have continuous positive airways pressure (CPAP) ventilation will not be at increased risk of apnea, even during the first night after surgery.

Patients with cardiovascular disease

As a general rule a patient who is unable to climb two flight of stairs at normal speed without experiencing cardiovascular symptoms (angina or heart failure, dyspnea), who has had a cardiac event (infarction, revascularization) within the previous 3 months, or who has a serious unstable condition or serious limitation of activity should be postponed or cancelled for ambulatory, elective surgery. Exceptions may be made if the surgery is very minor or noninvasive.

Hypertension

Stable hypertension with resting values up to 180 mmHg systolic or 110 mmHg diastolic is usually acceptable for ambulatory care. Isolated systolic values of 180–200 mmHg may be acceptable in the elderly if the diastolic pressure is below 110 mmHg. Otherwise, patients with newly discovered hypertension or very high values or unstable high values should be evaluated and optimized before being scheduled for ambulatory care.

Angina pectoris

While old studies state a 5% risk of developing perioperative coronary infarction in any angina patient, this figure is probably lower and much more varied in present practice, depending upon the degree of angina, the type of surgery, and perioperative monitoring or care. Angina patients are usually acceptable for ambulatory care if the condition has been stable for 3 months and they do not have regular attacks during minor activities (i.e., light housework, walking short distances on the flat), during rest or during the night. In cases with such symptoms a cardiologic evaluation should be undertaken and the possibility of postponement or inpatient care raised. If the preoperative assessment indicates that invasive blood pressure measurements will be required peroperatively, the patient may be scheduled for inpatient rather than ambulatory care. Similarly, an indication for nitroglycerine infusion means inpatient status.

Previous coronary infarction

If the infarction occurred less than 3 months previously, the general rule is to consider inpatient status as there is an increased risk of postoperative arrhythmia in the 3 months after an infarction.

This rule may be evaluated individually in cases where the infarction was small and uneventful, where the patient's function is very good and stable, and where the surgery is minor. Patients with clear signs of previous infarction on ECG (strong Q waves precordially or in II+III+AvR) but with no indication of symptoms in their history should be referred to a cardiologist for preoperative evaluation of cardiac function, with echocardiogram and exercise test. If there is no sign of cardiac dysfunction and no symptoms, patients with asymptomatic suspected previous infarction may be planned for ambulatory care in the same way as a stable angina patient with minor symptoms.

Previous revascularization

Patients should generally be postponed for 3 months after a revascularization procedure, in the same way as those who have had a coronary infarction, and be re-evaluated against the normal criteria for heart failure or angina. With successful revascularization and subsequent good clinical function, one should be aware of the risk of recurrence of symptoms and instability, which increase at 6 years or more after the procedure. A dedicated program for perioperative anticoagulation should be planned for revascularized patients (see later).

Heart failure

Patients with unstable and progressing heart failure and symptoms of dyspnea at rest or during minor indoor activities should not, as a general rule, be scheduled for ambulatory care. Typically the dyspnea with heart failure is worst while lying flat and improves when upright. Evaluation of the basic causes of heart failure should be taken into consideration: coronary artery disease, previous infarction, cardiomyopathy, valvular heart disease (see later), and arrhythmia. In some cases the condition may be improved by preoperative optimization 1–2 weeks before planned surgery. This may include angiotensin-converting enzyme (ACE) inhibitors, diuretics, and perhaps beta-blockers introduced carefully over a period of weeks.

Heart valve dysfunction

With heart valve (aortic or mitral) insufficiency, the feasibility of ambulatory care should be assessed according to the patient's level of function in keeping with the general rules (see above) regarding heart failure. Stenotic failures increase risk, even if symptoms are moderate. For any surgery that is invasive or requires general or major regional anesthesia, patients with aortic stenosis or mitral stenosis with functional limitation upon ordinary activity should be referred for cardiologic evaluation.

Patients with arrhythmia, heart block, or a pacemaker

Causes of arrhythmia should be checked and corrected if possible (e.g., thyrotoxicosis, aberrant atrioventricular bundles, and electrolyte abnormalities). Ventricular ectopic beats or episodes of asymptomatic unsustained tachyarrhythmias are not contraindications to ambulatory care. Patients with total atrioventricular (AV) block or patients with intermittent AV block and any history of fainting should be evaluated prior to all elective surgery for a pacemaker. Patients with an indwelling pacemaker or intracardiac defibrillator (ICD) with stable function (this should be verified!) and a stable clinical condition may have ambulatory surgery. Plans should be set in place for the proper use of electrocauterization and access to a device to program or control the pacemaker (magnet) should be considered.

Anticoagulated patients

These patients should be evaluated on a case-by-case basis by weighing the risk of short-term (from one to a few days) reduction or cessation of anticoagulation therapy against the risk of, and consequences of, bleeding as a result of the surgical procedure planned.

The first general rule is that patients should remain on their anticoagulation therapy as usual as long as there is a sound medical indication for it. There are exceptions for those types of surgery where bleeding may occur and be exacerbated by anticoagulation therapy.

Most surgery can be carried out on patients on low-dose *acetylsalicylic acid* prophylaxis without major problems due to bleeding. However, the hematomas may be a little more evident and the risk of increased blood loss following surgical accidents (e.g., unintentional rupture of a major vessel) may be increased. For these reasons, and also because the danger of stopping this prophylaxis for a few days is usually negligible, this drug is normally stopped for 4 days before the surgery and reinstated as soon as hemostasis is assured.

With *modern antiplatelet therapy* the indication for anticoagulation therapy is usually stronger (e.g., recent revascularization, mechanical heart valve) and the dosing strategy should be discussed with both hematologist and surgeon.

Similar individual strategies should be made for patients on *warfarin*. Most surgery can be carried out with an international normalized ratio (INR) value of 2 or less. However, care should be taken to minimize the period of reduced anticoagulation for conditions such as: atrial fibrillation, previous thromboembolic disease or episode, mechanical heart valve (in particular the mitral valve with low pressure and highly increased risk of thrombosis), and heart failure with an ejection fraction of less than 30%. A suggested regime for cases where there is a high risk of thromboembolism is to stop the warfarin 3–4 days prior to surgery, monitor the INR one to three times preoperatively, and institute a daily tailored dose of low-molecular-weight heparin (LMWH) once the INR is below 2.5. Similarly, postoperatively reinstate warfarin as soon as possible, supplemented by LMWH until the INR values are acceptable.

Anticoagulated patients will always have a higher than normal risk of developing *spinal hematomas* after spinal or epidural puncture, therefore these methods should only be used if there is a strong indication for them.

Obese patients

In developed and developing countries the total number and percentage of obese people in the population are increasing, as is their life expectancy. Ambulatory care is evolving for bariatric procedures of medium invasiveness (e.g., gastric banding or laparoscopic gastrectomy and bypass, see Chapter 5) in some places; although obese patients do present for all kinds of surgery, not just bariatric, and their suitability for ambulatory care needs to be assessed as for the population in general. Although the obese have reduced physiologic reserves, both cardiovascular and respiratory, obesity per se is not usually a major risk factor or reason for being turned down for ambulatory care. Rather, nonacceptance has to do with the overall problems presented by obesity, namely the frequent co-morbidity, the type of surgery planned, as well as practical aspects such as weight limits on the operating table and trolleys.

The following co-morbidities are more frequent in the obese population: diabetes mellitus, hypertonia, gastroesophageal reflux, arthrosis and musculoskeletal pain, sleep apnea syndrome, and, in more severe cases, pulmonary hypoventilation and atelectasis or heart failure.

Body mass index (BMI) is the most common way of classifying obesity, although it is an underestimate for short people and an overestimate for those who are very tall, muscular or heavily built. Some definitions of weight and obesity are listed in Table 3.3.

Table 3.3. Definitions of weight and obesity

Different types of weight:	actual weight = total weight ideal weight = height÷100 (105 in women) lean weight = fat-free body mass corrected ideal weight = ideal weight + 20–40% (?) of difference from actual weight
Body mass index (BMI) = weight/(height × height)	$\leq 25\,kg \cdot m^{-2}$ normal $25–30\,kg \cdot m^{-2}$ overweight $\geq 30\,kg \cdot m^{-2}$ obese $>35\,kg \cdot m^{-2}$ morbidly obese $>55\,kg \cdot m^{-2}$ super morbidly obese

Source: GA Bray, Pathology of obesity. *Am J Clin Nutr* 1992;**55**:448S–494S.

A calculation may be done for the exact BMI, although a rough estimate can be obtained by taking the height (in cm) and subtracting 100 (105 for women), which gives the ideal weight (in kg). Add 50% to the ideal weight to get a BMI of 35 (lower limit for being morbidly obese), or add 100% to get a BMI of 55 (lower limit for being super morbidly obese).

As a rule of thumb:

- Super morbidly obese patients will not usually be candidates for anything other than minor ambulatory surgery
- Obese patients (i.e., BMI: 30–35 $kg{\cdot}m^{-2}$) may routinely be candidates for ambulatory surgery, being assessed in the same way as the normal population for other presenting conditions and co-morbidity
- Morbidly obese patients (i.e., BMI: 35–55 $kg{\cdot}m^{-2}$) should be considered as candidates, but the combination of other presenting conditions and the type of surgery planned may sometimes render them unsuitable

If a procedure may be done with loco-regional anesthesia, this may support taking an ambulatory approach. If general anesthesia has to be used, spontaneous ventilation and a low or moderate duration of procedure will be favorable, as will minimized need for postoperative opioids. Obstructive sleep apnea syndrome may be a strong contraindication to ambulatory care (see above), whereas stable daily function may be a good indicator of the ambulatory potential of the morbidly obese, as with others.

Useful tests are ECG, spirometry, resting blood gas while breathing room air, pulmonary radiograph, and a functional test, such as walking a flight of stairs.

Diabetes mellitus

Diabetic patients may be unsuitable for ambulatory care if they have some of the more serious complications of prolonged diabetes, namely cardiovascular disease, kidney failure, neuropathy, and morbid obesity. It is important to check out these conditions in diabetic patients.

As to the diabetes per se, it is usually compatible with ambulatory care if the patient is otherwise stable and well regulated. However, if there is any doubt about an insulin-dependent patient's psychosocial competence to handle an unstable and often somewhat more variable blood sugar at home after same-day discharge, the threshold should be low for admitting them to inpatient care.

Important tests will be fasting blood sugar and the HbA1 to check for stability of blood sugar control (values above 9–10 indicate poor control). Further checks on signs of dehydration or acidosis should be made. If ambulatory care seems feasible, general advice to these patients is to behave as usual on the day before surgery: ordinary food, ordinary activity, ordinary dosing of antidiabetic medication, including insulin. On the morning of surgery the patient is advised to skip all antidiabetic drugs, to consume no food or drink, and to come to the hospital for a blood sugar test when the unit opens. It is usually wise to place these patients second or third on the list, thus allowing time for blood sugar measurement and appropriate planning.

Alcohol or drug abuse

From a medical point of view most of these patients can be ambulatory provided they do not have any serious accompanying condition which in itself excludes ambulatory care. It is important to ascertain that their nutritional status as well as vitamins and electrolytes are well controlled. A laboratory screen for hemoglobin, liver function, kidney function, electrolytes, blood-borne disease [human immunodeficiency virus (HIV), hepatitis] may be appropriate.

These patients should be advised to reduce or stop their abuse in a controlled way before planned surgery, but if this is impossible a more realistic approach is often to establish a stable pattern of abuse during the weeks and days before surgery.

The psychosocial situation of these patients is highly relevant to their suitability for ambulatory care. If there is any doubt about whether they or their carers at home will be able to handle pain treatment or any signs of complication appropriately, they should be referred as inpatients or to a hospital-hotel with proper monitoring.

Bodybuilders are a special group of drug abusers, who may be using drugs such as corticosteroids, insulin, and amphetamine-like drugs regularly. These patients may be treated by the ambulatory service, but an individualized regimen of peroperative medication substitution and precautions should be set in place. If possible these patients should be informed of the dangers of their drug practice (thrombosis, mental disturbance, cardiomyopathy, etc.) and persuaded well in advance of the surgery to stop or reduce the use of such drugs.

Other regular medication

Other regular medications are not usually an obstacle to ambulatory care, but the underlying disease may be.

The general rule for all medications needed by and indicated for a patient is to continue as usual, including any morning dose, which should be taken with a sip of water at least 1 hour prior to the scheduled start of anesthesia. Some exception apply to this general rule:

- *Anticoagulants* (see Anticoagulated patients)
- *Antidiabetics and insulin* (see Diabetes mellitus)
- *Oral contraceptives.* Estrogen-containing pills may increase the risk of thrombosis slightly, and the general rule is to advise the patient to stop this medication for 3–4 weeks prior to surgery and to use alternative methods of contraception for that period. This rule is not absolute and may be considered together with other risk factors for thrombosis, such as obesity, smoking, own or family history of venous thrombosis, planned prolonged or extended surgery, or use of a tourniquet. Also, the risk of an inadvertent pregnancy due to an unstable psychosocial situation or problems with alternative methods of contraception should be considered.
- *Angiotensin blockers.* These may sometimes create difficulties in maintaining a blood pressure adequate for organ perfusion when combined with general anesthesia and especially spinal or epidural anesthesia. Textbooks and reviewers differ in their advice on whether to stop these agents. A pragmatic view to take is that if the patient needs an ACE inhibitor for heart failure, their need will persist in the perioperative phase and the drug should be continued. If, however, the drug is used to control hypertension, it may be appropriate to skip the medication on the evening before surgery and/or the morning of surgery, and to control the event of hypertension with beta-blocker or other antihypertensives when or as needed.

Some drugs should certainly NOT be stopped or reduced, maybe even being reinforced during the perioperative phase:

- *Anti-asthmatics.* These drugs, sprays, and aerosols are often used intermittently and only during bad periods. If the patient is prescribed such drugs, it may be appropriate to advise taking them prophylactically, starting the day before surgery and then again on the morning of surgery, and to bring their spray or aerosol to the hospital so that they can take an extra dose just before the start of anesthesia.

- *Beta-blockers.* The benefit of starting beta-blockers in at-risk patients prior to major surgery remains controversial. However, there is no debate about the potential harmful effects of stopping beta-blockers just before surgery. Therefore patients should be asked specifically if they have taken their beta-blockers as normal.
- *Statins, cholesterol-lowering agents.* The evidence of problems caused by cessation of such medication is not as strong as that for beta-blockers, but there is good documentation of the potential benefits of continuing these drugs perioperatively. These drugs seem to have an anti-inflammatory effect that is beneficial for cardiovascular risk.

Psychiatric patients, patients with cognitive dysfunction or disabilities

These patients usually benefit from having as short and uneventful stay in the hospital environment as possible, as they are usually distressed by anything disrupting their normal routine and by any change in carer. Thus, if they can receive proper care after same-day discharge, they should be assigned to ambulatory care. They should receive all their normal medication until the start of anesthesia, perhaps with additional anxiolytic. It may be wise to make an appointment at their place of residence to ascertain whether a safe anxiolytic (i.e., benzodiazepine) should be given before they leave for the hospital, and also whether it would be appropriate to apply a local anesthetic pad for pain-free intravenous cannulation.

Acute disease

Ambulatory surgery should be planned at least one or two days in advance; thus, any acute need for surgery does not fit within this frame. Also, acute disease often implies an unstable physiology with pain, fluid balance disturbance, bleeding, and so on. Sometimes the diagnosis is unknown and often some postoperative observation of symptom progression is needed. A pragmatic approach may be taken if surgery fits in with the organization of the ambulatory unit. For instance, a broken leg or arm may be scheduled for surgery the next day with same-day discharge. Also non-severe abdominal pain may be scheduled for laparoscopy and cysts or abscesses for puncture, with potential for same-day discharge.

Pregnancy

Elective surgery and modern anesthesia have not been shown to pose any significant risk for either mother or child during pregnancy. That said, there is general concern for any procedure in this situation, especially exposure to chemical or physical stimuli with potential teratogenic effects in the first trimester and any stimulation that may initiate contractions and premature birth in the last trimester. Some modern painkillers [e.g., nonsteroidal anti-inflammatory drugs (NSAIDs), cyclooxygenase II (COX-II) inhibitors, glucocorticoids] are not approved for use during the first trimester. Thus, depending on its indication, most women will wait for their surgery. If there is a good indication for surgery (suspected malignancy, problematic symptoms, condition deteriorating if left untreated), an operation and appropriate anesthetic may be given during any phase of pregnancy, the preference being for the second trimester if selection of timing is an option. Whether surgery should be ambulatory or not will depend not on the pregnancy per se but on the patient's general condition and co-morbidities.

Breastfeeding patients

Breastfeeding is fully compatible with any surgery or anesthetic; this also applies to the ambulatory setting as long as the usual selection criteria are fulfilled. However, the patient should be warned against the regular use of benzodiazepines and codeine in the perioperative setting as these drugs may accumulate to dangerous levels in milk from some patients [21].

Other reasons for not being classified an ASA I or II patient

For most of the conditions in this section the patient will be eligible for ambulatory surgery if he or she is well functioning in daily life and if their condition is stable and appropriately treated.

Kidney disease

It is important to do a full laboratory work-up of these patients including hemoglobin, electrolytes, creatinine, urea, and blood gas. Low hemoglobin and high potassium are particularly important to identify. Dialysis patients should be dialyzed the day before surgery and a fresh set of laboratory results obtained on the day of surgery. Any anatomical abnormalities that have implications for instrumentation and practical handling should be noted on the chart: single kidney, hypertrophic kidney or urine collecting system, transplanted kidney, or abnormalities in the external urine outlet or genitalia.

Liver disease

A full laboratory screen is important, including liver enzymes [alanine transaminase (ALAT), aspartate transaminase (AST), and gamma glutamyl transpeptidase (GGT)], and even more importantly tests on liver function such as albumin, INR, and bilirubin. Anatomical issues may also be significant: is the liver large or fragile or is there any suspicion of esophageal varices? (avoid gastric tubing!). In cases of previous or ongoing hepatitis a full screen for viral (A, B, C) antigens and antibodies should be made, as should tests for HIV. If there is any chance that a blood-borne infection is present, it should be documented on the chart.

Thyroid disorders

These may be anatomical, namely an overt goiter that may cause airway problems. A radiograph (anterior and lateral projections) or computed tomography (CT) scan of the neck should be undertaken where there is the possibility of a displaced or compressed upper airway. Disorders of metabolism present more frequently than anatomical complications. Hyperthyroidism should be corrected before elective surgery; otherwise arrhythmia and unpredictable anesthetic drug dosing may result. Thyroid hormone replacement therapy should be instituted to achieve stable and appropriate levels in patients with hypothyroidism.

Rheumatoid arthritis, Bechterew disease (ankylosing spondylitis), and other rheumatic conditions

These patients will usually be eligible for ambulatory care if they have no other major co-morbidity. These patients generally have potential airway or intubation problems and require special anesthetic consideration, issues that usually are not relevant to the decision to schedule for ambulatory or inpatient care. It is appropriate to assess neck mobility and document the result on the chart; patients with a stiff neck should have a radiograph to document upper neck function. The indication to order a radiograph depends on the worst case scenario; for example, suspicion that the patient cannot be ventilated by mask, or that they may need intubation or require muscle relaxants.

Chest stiffness, ease of ventilation by laryngeal mask (LMA), and spine calcification (in case spinal anesthesia is required) should be checked. With nonspecific rheumatoid symptoms or neuromuscular complaints, ambulatory care is usually feasible. It is sensible to ask the patient to list drugs they cannot tolerate and to spend time reassuring them that non-specific symptoms are not worsened by having an anesthetic.

Neurologic diseases

For specified neurologic diseases ambulatory care is usually well tolerated, but it is important to document any paresis and discuss the anesthetic with the patient. Regional anesthesia and the implications of neural blockade for neurologic symptoms should be discussed thoroughly with the patient preoperatively. Uneventful regional anesthesia has not been shown to cause any deterioration in neurologic symptoms, but the topic may still arise for discussion postoperatively, which is better done preoperatively.

Myasthenic patients should continue with their ordinary medication and a fail-safe mechanism instituted for documenting the condition on the patient's chart to inform the anesthetist on the day of surgery of the patient's status.

Patients with epilepsy

Patients with epilepsy are usually eligible for ambulatory care, not least because most general anesthetics have anti-epileptic action in the perioperative phase. Patients who have frequent convulsions in spite of prophylaxis (which should always be continued pre- and perioperatively) may still be scheduled for ambulatory care, provided they are returning to an environment on the day of surgery (parents, spouse, specialized institution) where convulsions can be handled adequately.

Patients with allergy

Patients with allergies may be admitted for ambulatory care with known allergenic triggers and the severity of symptoms documented. It is important to ask patients about specific allergy symptoms (rash, mucous membrane secretions, airway obstruction), as many patients perceive drug side-effects to be allergies. Known examples of misconception are diarrhea after antibiotics, gastric acid secretion or pain after nonsteroidal anti-inflammatory drugs (NSAIDS), or vasovagal symptoms following local anesthesia.

Problems with previous anesthetics or with anesthesia in close family

It is important here to recognize unexplained jaundice (inhalational-anesthetic-associated hepatitis?), malignant hyperthermia, and cholinesterase deficiencies (prolonged duration of suxamethonium or mivacurium). These patients may still be treated in the ambulatory setting, but it is important to be aware of potential problems and diagnoses made prior to surgery.

It is important for the anesthetist to ascertain whether the patient has experienced nausea or vomiting, strong pain, or delayed emergence following a previous general anesthetic, although these problems are more innocent than those described above. More serious are reports of previous awareness, which should be carefully documented and require dedicated planning and communication with the patient.

Preoperative information

Preoperative information provided by the patient

It is very useful if the patient fills in a standard self-administered questionnaire prior to ambulatory surgery. This may save time when clerking the patient's health status, it ensures that important areas of general health are covered, and it gives the patient an opportunity to provide information in their own environment and at their own speed. It is most efficient if this is completed prior to surgical evaluation for the procedure, but it may also be valuable to repeat the process on the morning of surgery, to find out whether anything has been forgotten or there is any change in status. Having the patient sign the form gives it medicolegal status, should the patient later claim that the doctor forgot, did not hear, or had no time to listen to important issues. Typical areas of discussion are allergies and loose teeth; if the patient has ticked "no" on the signed form, it is hard for them to claim later that the hospital is to blame for not collecting relevant risk information in the case of a broken tooth or anaphylaxis. In some countries such a patient signature is mandatory and may also be coupled with a statement that the patient has received appropriate information about the procedure and its potential risks.

A patient form should be modified by and tailored to every unit, and a list of potential issues is listed below. It is wise to keep the form relatively short (one page is best), to have simple "yes" or "no" questions, to have space for extra information the patient may wish to provide, and to have an open question about anything else the patient wants to inform the unit about their health.

Example of a self-evaluation questionnaire for ambulatory surgery patients

Tick either "yes" or "no" to each question. If yes, then specify with short text or be prepared for more questions on the issue from the doctor/nurse.
   Have you had any of the following conditions or diseases:

1. Heart illness, vascular illness, fainting, or hypertension?
2. Lung disease, asthma or airway disease?
3. Diabetes?
4. Rheumatoid arthritis or other arthritis?
5. Hepatitis/HIV?
6. Allergy?
7. Tendency for bleeding or proneness to get blue spots (skin hematoma)?
8. Problems with teeth, opening the mouth, or moving the neck?
9. Do you smoke?
10. Are you, or could you be, pregnant or lactating?
11. Have you had general or regional anesthesia before?
12. Any problems with previous anesthesia?
13. Are there any problems with anesthesia in your family?
14. Have you stayed in hospital before?
15. Do you use any regular drugs? If yes, which ones and at what dose?

16. Do you use alcohol more than average?

17. Do you have any temporary health problem now?

18. Is there anything else you would like to tell us about your health?

19. My height is . . . . and my weight is approximately . . . .

I confirm that I have read through the form and that the information I have provided is correct.

Date . . . .

Signature . . . .

Preoperative information obtained by the physician

This is a somewhat more detailed list, which should been checked preoperatively for all patients by health personnel before the induction of anesthesia. The optimal situation is for the list to be sent beforehand by the patient's general practitioner to the ambulatory unit together with the patient's booking for potential surgery. If this is not possible, this information can be collected when the patient attends for preoperative surgical evaluation, when the list can be completed by the surgeon or by a nurse; the third opportunity to gather this information is if the patient is sent for a preoperative anesthetic consult.

The idea of having a detailed list is not necessarily that all issues should be commented upon, but that all issues have been checked. The documentation of a check may very well conclude with a phrase such as, "The patient is otherwise (apart from surgical indication) healthy and well functioning, takes no drugs, and has no known allergies."

List of health issues to be checked

If positive, state the degree and severity of symptoms and also document whether the condition is stable, unstable, improving, or deteriorating:

1. Hypertension, heart disease, thrombosis, breast pain, irregular heart rate, swollen legs

2. Asthma, chronic obstructive pulmonary disease (COPD), other pulmonary disease (ask the patient to bring their drugs in on day of surgery)

3. Tendency to bleed, bruises easily

4. Diabetes (ask patient to bring in their drugs, dosing and measurement equipment)

5. Hypo/hyperthyroidism

6. Repeated infections or contagious infections, such as hepatitis, HIV

7. Gastric/duodenal ulcer; reflux disease or acidic vomit

8. Airway obstruction, sleep apnea, loud snoring

9. Previous deep venous thrombosis, lung emboli, or family tendency to thrombosis

10. Epilepsy, migraine, stroke, transient ischemic attack (TIA), paralysis, or other conditions of the central nervous system

11. Cancer

12. Rheumatoid arthritis or other musculoskeletal disease

13. Allergy to drugs, latex, pollen, food, or anything else
14. Special diseases in the family
15. Previous hospital admissions; previous visits or admissions to hospitals abroad (any risk of methicillin-resistant *Staphylococcus aureus*?)

Drug history
1. What drugs does the patient take?
2. Drugs not tolerated by the patient (what is nature of intolerance?)
3. Is the patient on anticoagulation therapy?

Anesthesia and surgery
1. Has the patient had general or regional anesthesia before?
2. Were there any problems with previous anesthetics?
3. Is there a family history of anesthetic problems? (e.g. malignant hyperthermia, abnormal duration of suxamethonium or mivacurium)
4. Has the patient experienced nausea or vomiting after previous general anesthesia?

Other questions
1. Does the patient have false teeth, prosthetic teeth, or loose teeth?
2. Does the patient have problems with mouth opening or neck bending (backwards)?
3. Does the patient smoke? If so, how much, and is there any COPD?
4. Does the patient have a previous or current history of alcohol, tablet, or narcotic abuse?
5. Does patient have a chaperone to stay with him/her until the day after surgery?

Clinical examination
- Document patient's weight and height
- Document signs of infections or other intercurrent disease
- Document patient's blood pressure and heart rate (if irregular, take an ECG)
- Cardiopulmonary auscultation
- Assess level of function: can the patient climb two flights of stairs?

Important written supplemental information
- Copy of: hospital reports and specialist evaluations
- Copies of radiography, laboratory and ECG results

Preoperative information given to the patient

It is important that the patient receives written and oral information about the practicalities, potential risks, and problems that may occur before, during, and after surgery. It is often practical to give much of this information before the patient is admitted to the unit and then to repeat it just before they are discharged, and then to supplement with a detailed report of the surgery and any special precautions required.

There are at least three principles to consider when deciding how much detail should be given concerning potential side-effects and complications (events):

1. Any frequent event should be mentioned, e.g., nausea, tiredness, disturbed sleep. The term "frequent" is contentious: some say that anything occurring with an incidence of 2–4% is frequent; others will draw the line at 10–20%. Some argue that it is not mandatory to inform patients about events that are almost always inevitable (e.g., wound pain on movement).

2. Any potentially serious event should be mentioned, even if it is relatively infrequent. For instance, if the risk of major disability is 0.2%, most patients would like to know. It can be argued that if the risk of a serious event is very low (e.g., a risk of bleeding to death with tonsillectomy of 1 in 10 000), it may frighten the patient unduly to mention this specifically. A better approach may be to state that serious bleeding occurs very rarely, and then only specify the outcome if the patient asks.

3. More thorough information is warranted if the planned procedure is totally elective. If the procedure is indicated absolutely (e.g., removal of a breast cancer tumor), the benefit to the patient definitely outweighs any minor risk of having the procedure, and there may be an argument for not frightening the patient with knowledge about rare and dangerous complications. Nevertheless, it may be wise to inform the patient about the fairly frequent side-effects encountered to help them form a realistic expectation of the outcome. Elective cosmetic procedures, such as breast implants in a young healthy girl, fall at the other end of the spectrum. It may be appropriate to inform such patients about the low (but still relevant) risk of having chronic pain, loss of sensation or hyperalgesia in some areas, and problems with lactation to enable them to make a fully informed decision about having the procedure.

An example of standard information is given in the following box for a procedure that is indicated to improve a patient's quality of life (e.g., hernia repair, varicose veins), and is not life-saving. The information can be adapted to individual institutions, patients, procedures, and medicolegal situations. Surgeons should supply their specific information, either separately or integrated with information about anesthesia and logistics into one information "package."

Plan for anesthesia

Anesthesia in some form or another will be needed for your planned operation. For some surgical procedures local or regional anesthesia may be used, whereas for others general anesthesia is recommended. Sometimes we use a combination of these methods. Any special requests you may have for the type of anesthesia may be discussed with the anesthesiologist beforehand. Sometimes the choice between different types of anesthesia and the practical setup also depend on the following issues:

- Whether you have other diseases
- Whether you have any allergies
- Whether you are on any medications or are using drugs
- Whether you smoke

- Whether you are pregnant
- Whether you bleed or bruise easily
- Whether you have had a previous thrombosis
- Whether you have problems with mouth opening or neck movements
- Whether you are normally physically fit or not
- Whether you drink more than the recommended levels of alcohol or have any other abuse problems
- Whether you have any special issues with your teeth: prosthetic, loose, etc.
- Previous anesthetic history
- Whether someone in your close family has had problems with an anesthetic

Logistics
On the day of surgery you should not eat anything or have milk products in the six hours prior to admittance. You should not drink any clear fluids in the two hours prior to admittance, although an exception to this rule may be your ordinary morning medication, which you should take as normal with a sip of water, unless you receive different instructions (there are special rules for antidiabetic medications, insulin, and anticoagulants).

You should have a shower or wash in the morning, wear comfortable leisure clothes, and do not apply make-up. It may be wise to bring a paper, book, or music player, although we do have some of these in our waiting facility. You should arrange for someone responsible (who is able to make a phone call and make decisions) to be with you at home until the following morning and preferably have someone to escort you home after discharge.

Risks and side-effects
You should be aware that every type of surgery and anesthetic carries a risk for side-effects and complications. The most usual after a general anesthesia is temporary tiredness and a change in sleeping pattern and quality for the first one to two nights. We will give you prophylaxis and treatment to minimize pain and to avoid nausea, but you may experience these problems anyway. If so, you will receive supplemental drugs as needed.

Everyone has a right to information about what they will experience during their stay in the ambulatory surgery unit. Everyone who is scheduled to have an anesthetic will have a consultation with an anesthesiologist or nurse-anesthetist before they receive any medication or anesthesia is induced. It may be wise to note down beforehand any particular issues you want to discuss. You are also welcome to contact us in advance if there are things about your anesthetic you want to discuss.

Rare complications associated with anesthesia may be:

- Headache after spinal or epidural anesthesia. This is a fairly rare event (less than 5%), usually mild, and never lasts for more than a few days. If strong, there are treatment options
- Minor, transient pain localized in the back after spinal or epidural needle puncture
- Temporary cessation of micturition after spinal or epidural anesthesia (more frequent in elderly men)
- Tingling and changed sensation for one to two days in an area that has been anesthetized with local or regional anesthetic
- Stiffness or slight aching in the muscles for one to two days after some particular types of general anesthesia

- Allergic reactions to anesthetic drugs or to adjuvants (dressings, fluids, antibiotics). Such reactions may rarely be serious, but will be stopped by the anesthetic staff
- Sore throat or hoarse voice for a few days after having a plastic tube inserted for breathing with general anesthesia
- Temporary soreness and discoloration (which may last for weeks) at the site of intravenous access for infusion of drugs and fluids
- Injuries to your teeth, especially if these are already loose or weak
- Heart or lung complications, especially if you have existing cardiopulmonary or vascular disease
- Deep venous thrombosis in a limb may occur during your stay in the unit or emerge after discharge

Appendix 3.1: The ASA (American Society of Anaesthesiologists) classification of general preoperative health

Original version

ASA I: A normal healthy patient

ASA II: A patient with mild systemic disease

ASA III: A patient with severe systemic disease

ASA IV: A patient with severe systemic disease that is a constant threat to life

ASA V: A moribund patient who is not expected to survive without the operation

ASA VI: A declared brain-dead patient whose organs are being removed for donor purposes

Short updated version

This is based on the original setup, where an important aspect was NOT to make long, official detailed lists of conditions and diseases. As such lists may always be the subject of discussion and may result in reluctance to use the score (when the list is not to hand), it may be wise to have the ASA classification very roughly and robustly defined for everyone to remember and everyone to use. Problems remain with the original version in that it talks only about systemic disease and does not include severe single-organ disease; furthermore, there is no classification for "moderate" disease, i.e., disease between mild and severe.

Thus, this modified short version is a pragmatic approach taken from many sources and my own clinical practice:

ASA class I: Healthy patient (i.e., nothing remarkable in the history or physical examination)

ASA class II: Healthy patient, but with remarks noted about health or defined disease (i.e., normal vital functions retained in daily life)

ASA class III: Patient with moderate clinical illness (significant disease and/or some disability, usually limiting vital functions and daily life)

ASA class IV: Severely ill patient with serious limitation in vital functions

ASA class V: Patient with an immediately life-threatening condition

Extended version

As it will be useful to set some examples of classification this is frequently done in the literature, and it is also useful to have a unified opinion on classification of some very frequent situations and disease states. This is a more detailed list, again fairly pragmatic and from many sources:

ASA 1: Healthy patient. No organic, physiologic, biochemical, or psychiatric disorder. The surgical condition (i.e., which is planned for surgery) is localized and results in no general systemic disorders.

ASA 2: Healthy patient with remarks. These patients have a moderate organic disease or disturbance, or a condition with limited physiological reserve capacity. Examples: Age >80 years or newborns <3 months age after term delivery. Patients who smoke more than five cigarettes per day. Patients with uncomplicated (noninsulin-dependent) diabetes mellitus. Patient with stable and uncomplicated hypertension. Patient with obesity and no other disease.

ASA 3: Patient with moderate clinical illness. These patients have some significant organic or psychiatric disease or physiologic disturbance, which results in defined limitations of function. Examples: diabetes mellitus requiring insulin treatment or organic complications, moderate to severe heart disease or lung disease, angina pectoris, previous myocardial infarction, chronic obstructive pulmonary disease with limitation in daily life.

ASA 4: Severely ill patient. These patients have life-threatening organic disease. Examples: malignant hypertension, previous myocardial infarction (within the previous 6 months), advanced dysfunction of liver, kidney or lungs; established heart failure, unstable angina, recent stroke or subarachnoid bleeding.

ASA 5: Patient with an immediately life-threatening condition. These are patients with a less than 50% chance of survival if left untreated. Examples: patients in hypovolemic shock, deeply comatose patients with airway or breathing problems.

References

1. Gudimetta V, Smith I. Pre-operative screening and selection of adult day surgery patients. In: Lemos P, Jarrett P, Philip B, eds. *Day Surgery – Development and Practice*, London: IAAS, 2006: 125–38.

2. Trondsen E, Mjaland O, Raeder J, Buanes T. Day-case laparoscopic fundoplication for gastro-oesophageal reflux disease. *Br J Surg* 2000;**87**:1708–11.

3. Mjaland O, Raeder J, Aasboe V, et al. Outpatient laparoscopic cholecystectomy. *Br J Surg* 1997;**84**:958–61.

4. Levy BS, Luciano DE, Emery LL. Outpatient vaginal hysterectomy is safe for patients and reduces institutional cost. *J Minim Invasive Gynecol* 2005;**12**:494–501.

5. An HS, Simpson JM, Stein R. Outpatient laminotomy and discectomy. *J Spinal Disord* 1999;**12**:192–6.

6. Hval K, Thagaard KS, Schlichting E, Raeder J. The prolonged postoperative analgesic effect when dexamethasone is added to a nonsteroidal antiinflammatory drug (rofecoxib) before breast surgery. *Anesth Analg* 2007;**105**:481–6.

7. Ruiz-Deya G, Davis R, Srivastav SK, et al. Outpatient radical prostatectomy: impact of standard perineal approach on patient outcome. *J Urol* 2001;**166**:581–6.

8. Krywulak SA, Mohtadi NG, Russell ML, Sasyniuk TM. Patient satisfaction with inpatient versus outpatient reconstruction of the anterior cruciate ligament: a randomized clinical trial. *Can J Surg* 2005;**48**:201–6.

9. Lewis RA, Buss DD. Outpatient shoulder surgery: a prospective analysis of a perioperative protocol. *Clin Orthop Relat Res* 2001;**390**:138–41.

10. Chattar-Cora D, Okoro SA, Barone CM. Abdominoplasty can be performed successfully as an outpatient procedure with minimal morbidity. *Ann Plast Surg* 2008;**60**:349–52.

11. Sahai A, Symes A, Jeddy T. Short-stay thyroid surgery. *Br J Surg* 2005;**92**:58–9.

12. Gravningsbraten R, Nicklasson B, Raeder J. Safety of laryngeal mask airway and short-stay practice in office-based adenotonsillectomy. *Acta Anaesthesiol Scand* 2009;**53**:218–22.

13. Ansell GL, Montgomery JE. Outcome of ASA III patients undergoing day case surgery. *Br J Anaesth* 2004;**92**:71–4.

14. Hannalah R. Pediatric issues for ambulatory surgery. In: Lemos P, Jarrett P, Philip B, eds. *Day Surgery – Development and Practice*, London: IAAS, 2006: 139–56.

15. Jonas DA. Parent's management of their child's pain in the home following day surgery. *J Child Health Care* 2003;**7**:150–62.

16. Hug M, Tonz M, Kaiser G. Parental stress in paediatric day-case surgery. *Pediatr Surg Int* 2005;**21**:94–9.

17. Canet J, Raeder J, Rasmussen LS, et al. Cognitive dysfunction after minor surgery in the elderly. *Acta Anaesthesiol Scand* 2003;**47**:1204–10.

18. Young T, Palta M, Dempsey J, et al. The occurrence of sleep-disordered breathing among middle-aged adults. *N Engl J Med* 1993;**328**:1230–5.

19. Lofsky A. Cases of sleep apnea syndrome. *Anesth Pt Safety Found Newsl* 2002;**17**:24–5.

20. Chung SA, Yuan H, Chung F. A systemic review of obstructive sleep apnea and its implications for anesthesiologists. *Anesth Analg* 2008;**107**:1543–63.

21. Berlin CM, Jr., Paul IM, Vesell ES. Safety issues of maternal drug therapy during breastfeeding. *Clin Pharmacol Ther* 2009;**85**:20–2.

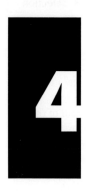

4 Pharmacology

For ambulatory anesthesia good knowledge of pharmacology is especially important. The case turnover is rapid and, in order to be discharged on the same day, patients should have a complete and clearheaded recovery with minimal side-effects. While the procedures usually are of short or intermediate duration, the surgical stimulation may still be strong at times, which calls for precise knowledge about how to adjust and time drug effects.

The relationship between a given dose and the observed effect may be divided as: (1) the relationship between dose and plasma level (pharmacokinetics) and (2) the relationship between plasma level and effect(s) (pharmacodynamics).

While we as clinical anesthesiologists are primarily interested in the effect, it is still useful to know the laws that dictate plasma concentration. Better understanding of plasma concentration will help us to achieve the desired effect level more precisely.

General aspects (see Figure 4.1)

Strongly hypnotic, analgesic, and anti-nociceptive drugs have to be lipid soluble in order to penetrate the blood–brain barrier and reach their target cells in the central nervous system (CNS), where they have their effect. Lipid solubility creates two problems: the drugs are also distributed extensively into all other cells and tissues, and they are not readily excreted through the kidneys. Their *distribution volume* may be calculated by dividing the dose by the plasma concentration.

Fortunately, the brain and spinal cord have a large blood supply and thus receive a high dose of drug initially after a bolus dose or at the start of a high-dose infusion/inhalation before other tissues "steal" a large number of the drug molecules. The infusion or inhalation has to be maintained at an appropriate level to compensate for the ongoing loss of drug into tissues that are abundant and not relevant to the anesthetic effect. The speed and amount of drug diffusion into different organs depend upon the blood flow to those organs, the plasma concentration (or partial pressure for inhalational agents), the concentration gradient between the blood and tissue, and drug solubility in the tissues.

Elimination of anesthetic drugs via the kidneys is not a prerequisite for the successful ending of anesthesia. Inhalational agents are excreted through exhalation and iv drugs are metabolized to water-soluble metabolites, which can be excreted renally. Many agents have been tested and successfully used for general anesthesia. The commonly used drugs discussed in this chapter have been chosen through an evolutionary process, to result in the selection of the best drugs that share some beneficial features: they have low toxicity, a low potential to induce anaphylactic reactions, high rate of metabolism, inactive metabolites, and are metabolized through a first-order reaction that ensures that a constant fraction is being metabolized all the time. In contrast to zero-order metabolism (in which a constant amount of drug

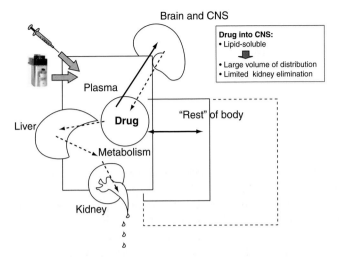

Brain and CNS

Drug into CNS:
• Lipid-soluble

• Large volume of distribution
• Limited kidney elimination

Plasma

Liver

Drug

"Rest" of body

Metabolism

Kidney

Figure 4.1. Anatomical model of anesthesia pharmacology.
An anesthetic drug is delivered to the plasma from a vaporizer (via the lungs) or intravenously as bolus injections or infusions. From plasma the drug will diffuse into the central nervous system (CNS), where the effects of sleep and anti-nociception (analgesia) are initiated. Simultaneously a large amount of drug diffuses into rest of the body. Also, the process of metabolism in the liver commences, to form a water-soluble, inactive metabolite which is excreted in the urine.

is metabolized per unit time), first-order mechanisms protect somewhat against unlimited accumulation with overdose. This is because metabolism increases as drug levels in the plasma accumulate. By constant continuous dosing the rate of elimination tends to (after 3–5 times the elimination half-life) equate to the rate of drug supply and the plasma level reaches a plateau.

For most drugs metabolism takes place in the liver. The maximum potential clearance of a liver-metabolized drug equates to the liver blood flow, which is about 1.5 liters per minute in an adult. *Clearance* is defined as the amount of blood that is fully cleaned of drug per unit time. For some drugs, such as propofol, there is extra-hepatic metabolism (enzymes in lung, gut, etc.), thus the clearance may be somewhat higher than liver blood flow. An even more efficient way of ensuring rapid drug elimination is to manufacture drugs that are eliminated by enzymes that are widespread throughout the body, thus enabling more extensive and liver-independent degradation. This is the case with remifentanil, which is degraded by tissue esterases very rapidly and extensively. There is also work in progress to develop propofol-like or benzodiazepine drugs with these characteristics in order to ensure their ultra-rapid metabolism.

Neuromuscular blocking agents and reversal agents do not need to be lipid soluble, because their receptors are on the surface of the muscle membranes and thus accessible to water-soluble drugs. Although some of these drugs are also partly degraded in the liver, they do not diffuse readily through membranes and into cells, thus their distribution volumes are lower than for lipid-soluble drugs.

Inhalational drugs: pharmacokinetics (Figure 4.2)

The metabolism of modern inhalational drugs is negligible and does not contribute quantitatively to the amount of drug in the body. It is the partial pressure of the agent that is responsible for the anesthetic effect, but at sea level at 1 atmosphere of pressure, the value in kPa will be the same as the percentage of the total (1 atm is approximately 100 kPa). Although this partial pressure will be correlated to concentration for individual agents, the agents differ in terms of solubility: high solubility means that a large number of

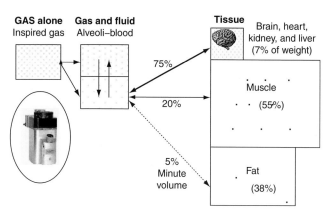

Figure 4.2. The gas molecules are delivered to the alveoli via the endotracheal tube, LMA, or mask and equilibrate (to equal partial pressure) with the lung blood. In a sleeping patient about 75% of the cardiac output will go to the brain, heart, kidney, and liver, which are only about 7% of the total body mass. 20% of the minute volume will go to the 55% of body mass which is muscle and 5% will go to fat. Thus the brain cells will fairly rapidly receive a large dose of drug, whereas the muscle and fat will continue to take up molecules for a very long time before equilibrium.

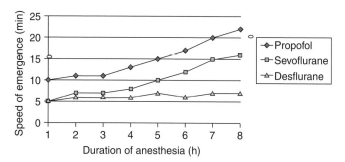

Figure 4.3. Speed of emergence (min) after different hypnotic, anesthetic agents have been given for standardized maintenance (x-axis) of general anesthesia over 1–8 h: a patient given propofol will wake up at 10 min after 1 h of anesthesia, and at 20 min after 7 h of anesthesia, whereas a patient given desflurane will wake up at 7 min after 7 h and at 5 min after 1 h.

molecules is needed in the blood or tissue in order to build up a given partial pressure and effect. The partial pressure of an inhalational agent in a patient is dictated by the amount the patient inhales, equilibration between alveoli and blood, the binding of drug molecules to fluid and cells, and duration of exposure. A low solubility in blood means a more rapid establishment of a high partial pressure by induction, and a more efficient exhalation at the end of anesthesia, thus a more rapid induction and emergence. Nitrous oxide, sevoflurane, and desflurane are fairly equal in this respect, whereas isoflurane, halothane, and enflurane are more soluble and slower. However, with sevoflurane (and also halothane) the speed of induction can be further increased by giving a very high concentration (overpressure) initially, whereas with desflurane and isoflurane high initial concentrations will be irritating (coughing, spasm) for the airways and not work clinically. Nitrous oxide is too weak to be fully anesthetic by itself, and is only useful as an adjuvant.

For procedures of 1–2 h in duration the *blood solubility* is the most important determinant of emergence speed, but with prolonged cases the *tissue solubility* and amount of gas dissolved in the tissue will be increasingly important. Nitrous oxide is the least tissue soluble and will be rapidly exhaled and cleared from the tissues, also by prolonged exposure. Desflurane is better than sevoflurane in this respect (i.e., less tissue soluble) and will result in a more rapid emergence after procedures lasting more than 2–3 h (Figure 4.3). The higher the amount of fat a patient has, the greater the amount of drug distributed in the tissues, thus emergence from sevoflurane may be slower even after as little as one hour of anesthesia.

Inhalational agents can be monitored in individual patients by end-tidal measurement, although this end-tidal concentration is not always exactly the same as the partial pressure in arterial blood. In all patients there will be a slight delay in the change of partial pressure in blood and a further delay in brain changes compared with alveolar changes. End-tidal values will be a little higher than blood and brain values during induction and a little lower during emergence. These discrepancies are exaggerated when a patient lies flat on an operating table and further when the patient is elderly, fat, or ventilated by overpressure. This is owing to alveolar shunting of blood through alveoli that are not ventilated and therefore not equilibrating with the alveolar gas. The discrepancy between brain and blood measurements may be in the range of 10–50%, most with prolonged procedures and least when positive end-expiratory pressure (PEEP) is used.

A hyper-dynamic circulation (high cardiac minute volume) will generally slow down the induction and emergence somewhat because the brain blood flow is auto-regulated and constant. A high cardiac output results in more wash-in or wash-out (emergence) of inhalational drug from other tissues, creating respectively a lower (induction) and higher (emergence) partial pressure of inhalational drug in mixed blood delivered to the CNS.

Hyperventilation may create a more efficient wash-in and wash-out of inhalational drugs in blood, but this effect will be counteracted by a decrease in arterial partial pressure of carbon dioxide (pCO_2) and subsequent cerebral vasoconstriction, which will slow down the shift of inhalational drug in to or out of the brain.

With a high flow of fresh gas into the ventilation system, the difference in partial pressure between inspiratory and expiratory alveolar gas will not be extensive; thus turning the vaporizer setting to 1 MAC (where MAC stands for minimum alveolar concentration) may be expected to deliver close to 1 MAC in end-alveolar gas with a fresh gas flow of 6–8 liters per minute. However, low-flow circular systems are encouraged for maintenance from economical and humidity/temperature regulation points of view. Then the changes in vaporizer setting may be quite misleading as to changes in alveolar and blood partial pressures, which will be much slower and smaller compared with changes in the vaporizer figures. The best is usually to either "overdose" with the vaporizer or, especially at end of the case, to increase the fresh gas flow in order to achieve a rapid change in alveolar concentration. In both cases the end-alveolar partial pressure (= end-alveolar % at 1 atm or 100 kPa) is a good monitor of what is going on, with some reservations as to aspects of alveolar and arterial discrepancies as discussed above.

The use of inhalational agents in different settings (i.e., different patient weights, fresh gas flow, ventilation, cardiac output) in terms of partial pressure changes in different parts of the body as a function of time may be simulated in programs such as the GasMan (www.gasmanweb.com).

Inhalational drugs: pharmacodynamics

The relationship between stable levels of an inhalational drug in blood as described by stable end-tidal values and the effect is very well established by the MAC concept, where 1 MAC is the partial pressure needed for 50% of patients to lie still on incision. In order to have 95% of patients lying still, a concentration of 1.3 MAC is needed. A MAC value may also be defined as the end-point at which 50% of the patients are asleep, i.e., MACsleep. MACsleep in 50% of patients is about 0.33 MAC for all the potent inhalational agents, and about 0.67 MAC for nitrous oxide. In order to have 95% of the patients asleep a further 30% should be added, thus MACsleep95 will be about 0.45 MAC for the potent agents. A value of 0.5 is easy to remember and calculate, and also provides a small safety margin. This figure is important practically, because the inhalational agents are often used in low concentration to ensure sleep, while opioid or loco-regional anesthesia may be used for analgesia and anti-nociception. Thus, in order to ensure patients stay safely asleep in 95% of cases, stable brain values of 1.0 kPa (or 1%) sevoflurane, 3 kPa desflurane, or 0.6 kPa isoflurane are needed. For nitrous oxide this value (50% of MAC + 30%) will be 90 kPa, which is impossible to give. Nevertheless, at 67% nitrous oxide may have a "hypnotic" contribution equal to that of 1 MACsleep50, which may be added to other inhalational drugs or hypnotics. The MAC of nitrous oxide means that it is used as an adjunct to the potent drugs, but the additive value of 67% nitrous oxide is slightly less than 1 MACsleep50 when used in children and with desflurane. For a 95% chance of being asleep with 67% nitrous oxide the concentration of sevoflurane should be 0.5%; of desflurane, 1.5%; and of isoflurane, 0.3%.

MAC may also be defined for amnesia. Although not very well characterized for inhalational agents, the value is lower than MACsleep. Thus if a patient is safely asleep on an inhalational agent alone there is no risk of awareness, and the patient may also be somewhat protected against awareness when they are very sleepy, just before they become fully asleep.

The potent inhalational agents are quite similar in their effect-versus-side-effect profile, but some differences exist at equipotent dosing. Desflurane has been shown to be less of a respiratory depressant than sevoflurane (and isoflurane) at equipotent concentrations [1]. When a high concentration of desflurane (1 MAC or more) is given without titration, the airway irritation may result in sympathetic stimulation leading to a rise in heart rate and blood pressure. The increase may be both substantial and dangerous as it can be misinterpreted as indicating too small an anesthetic effect, whereas in fact the opposite is the case. However, this sympathetic stimulation is never seen with desflurane given at less than 1 MAC, nor when any concentration above 1 MAC is introduced with gradual titration over a period of minutes. As to cardiovascular effects, isoflurane seems to be the strongest vasodilator whereas halothane seems to be the most cardiodepressive (at equipotency), with sevoflurane and desflurane being intermediate on both measures. Sevoflurane is regarded as safe for not being vasodilatory [potentially increasing the intracranial pressure (ICP)] in the brain when given at less than 1 MAC. All the potent inhalational agents have been shown to induce pre-conditioning, that is they will protect the cardiac cells somewhat against damage during episodes of hypoxemia.

The potent agents also provide some muscle relaxation, but a high dose level (2–3 MAC) is needed to keep the laryngeal muscles relaxed during intubation with inhalational agents alone.

Nitrous oxide has very minor respiratory depressant and cardiovascular effects, the latter partly due to a mild sympathetic stimulation, which counteracts the cardiodepression.

All the inhalational agents seem to have the potential to induce emesis postoperatively, at least when compared to propofol for maintenance.

Dynamic interactions with intravenous agents

The intravenous (iv) opioids and hypnotics will interact with inhalational agents, but somewhat differently according to the class of iv drug and type of effect. The clinical interactions are logical: combination of inhalational agent with an iv hypnotic will provide additive hypnotic effect, but not much more analgesic effect. Combination of an inhalational agent with an iv analgesic will provide additive analgesic effect, but only slightly increased hypnotic effect [2–4].

a. The MACsleep may be reduced for a given drug in a linear manner by adding increasing amounts of the hypnotics propofol or midazolam. With midazolam 0.1 mg/kg iv, MACsleep for a potent inhalational agent will be reduced by about 50%; similar results are achieved with a propofol plasma level of 1.5 µg/ml.

b. The MACsleep is reduced by only 10–20% after a 0.2 mg dose of fentanyl in the adult, corresponding to a target of 7–8 ng/ml remifentanil or an infusion of 0.3 µg/kg per minute. Some patients may be fully asleep on a high opioid dose alone, however individual variation is huge, thus an average reduction in MACsleep of 50% demands a very high dose of opioid (fentanyl 0.6 mg or other opioid in an equipotent dose) and the effect is unpredictable.

c. The MAC to achieve an analgesic effect will be reduced by 60% by a fentanyl dose of 0.2 mg, and by 75% by doubling this dose.

d. The MAC to achieve an analgesic effect will be reduced by hypnotics by 30–40% by adding midazolam (0.1 mg/kg bolus) or by a propofol plasma level of 1.5 ng/ml. The effect of adding further hypnotics iv is infra-additive. Nevertheless, very high (intoxicating) doses of hypnotics actually have an anti-nociceptive clinical action.

Intravenous drugs: pharmacokinetics

For iv drugs the plasma concentration is determined by administration, tissue distribution, and elimination. A physiological model may be used (Figure 4.1), although it is more practical for dosing and calculation to use a mathematical model, derived from plasma concentration measurements in volunteers or patients after defined dosing of drugs. The distribution and elimination of iv drugs after dosing follow logarithmic laws, and are well described in a three-compartment model as in Figure 4.4. The mathematical construct of V1 may be regarded as analogous to plasma plus the fluid and tissue very close to blood vessels, whereas V2 may be those parts of the body receiving an intermediate proportion of the cardiac output, while V3 is poorly circulated, including fat tissue.

A bolus dose will result in a very high initial plasma concentration (in V1), which subsequently diffuses into V2 and V3. Because both V2 and V3 receive drug down a high concentration gradient initially, the decline in concentration in both plasma and V1 is rapid, but then slows as V2 equilibrates with V1. The third compartment (V3) fills very slowly due to its lower perfusion with blood. Also, constant (in terms of fraction of plasma drug metabolized per unit time) metabolism will continue and is responsible for only a small fraction of the total decline in plasma concentration initially. An infusion is, in principle, multiple, very rapidly repeated small bolus administrations of a constant amount and at a constant interval. A stable infusion will create an initially quickly, and then slowly, increasing plasma level, that is not fully stable until 3–5 times the elimination half-life of the drug. Then all compartments (V1–V3) in the body are in diffusion equilibrium and the amount of drug metabolized is equal to the amount given per time unit if the concentration is steady. At this point a constant relationship is given for the time taken to reduce the

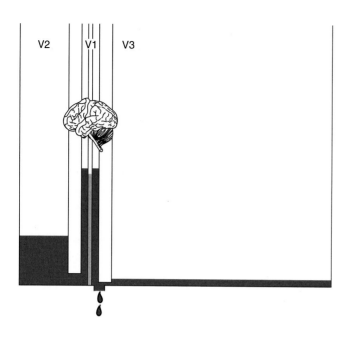

Figure 4.4. Mathematical three-compartment model with effect compartment embedded in volume 1 (V1). In the middle is V1, which receives drug and may be analogous to plasma and surrounding fluids. The level of black corresponds to drug concentration. From V1 there is good diffusion (a large opening) of drug into V2, which equilibrates with V1 within 10–30 min. A much slower diffusion takes place into V3 (a narrow opening), which is the larger part of the body and relatively poorly circulated. We may also note a constant "leakage" of drug from V1, which represents the clearance, inactivation, and/or excretion of the drug. The small grey compartment inside V1 is the CNS or effect compartment.

The level of drug (black; grey in the brain) is an example of simulation 10 min after a bolus dose of propofol (from Tivatrainer®).

plasma level of drug by 50% after cessation of dosing (the $T_{1/2}$ steady-state or $t^{1/2}_{beta/gamma}$), according to the formula:

$$T_{1/2} = V_D/\text{clearance} \times k$$

Clearance is defined as the amount of plasma fully cleared per unit time, and volume of distribution (V_D) is the volume needed to contain all the drug in the body (= total dose ÷ amount metabolized/excreted) if all tissues have the same drug concentration as plasma. For a 70-kg person a V_D of 5 liters (or 0.07 l/kg) means that the drug only stays in the plasma; a V_D of 70 liters (or 1 l/kg) means that the drug is evenly distributed at the same concentration as in plasma in all parts of the body; whereas a V_D of more than 70 liters or >1 l/kg means that the drug is present in higher mean concentrations outside the plasma (V1) than inside. For instance the "distribution volume" of propofol is more than 200 liters or 3 l/kg because propofol is highly lipid soluble and has a higher concentration in fat tissue than in plasma at equilibrium.

With most iv anesthetic drugs (except remifentanil, stable after 20–30 min) it takes more than 12–24 h to reach this level of steady-state by continued, stable dosing (Figure 4.5). Thus, for all cases of ambulatory iv anesthesia, the 50% reduction of plasma level by cessation of dosing, called $T_{1/2}$-context sensitive, will be given by the formula:

$$T_{1/2} = (V_D/\text{clearance} \times k_1) \div (\text{diffusion from V1 to V2} + \text{V3}) \times k_2$$

This diffusion is more extensive the shorter the period of drug administration, this time of administration is the "context" of this decline in plasma concentration as expressed in Figure 4.6.

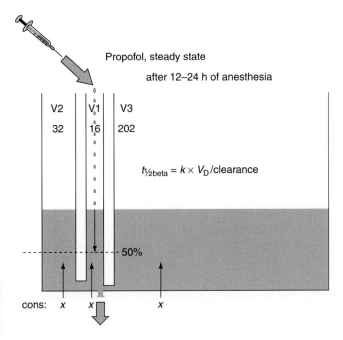

Propofol, steady state

after 12–24 h of anesthesia

V2
32

V1
16

V3
202

$t_{\frac{1}{2}beta} = k \times V_D / clearance$

50%

cons: x   x   x

Figure 4.5. Steady state picture of propofol in a 3-compartment model, 70 kg adult patient. Note that the volume of V2 and V3 are upgraded in order to contain propofol at the same concentration (x) as in plasma. In a pure anatomical model (total volume= 70 liters) the V2 would be 16 liters and propofol concentration 2x, whereas the V3 would be 38 liters and propofol concentration about 6x.

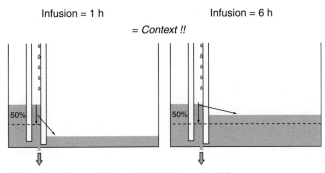

Infusion = 1 h   Infusion = 6 h

= Context !!

50%   50%

Same clearance – different distribution potential
→ Different $T_{1/2}$ related to "context"!

Figure 4.6. The same model as in Figure 4.5, but the propofol has been given for 1 h (left panel) or for 6 h (right panel). Note that in both cases the V2 is in equilibrium with the V1, but the V3 is "filled" less after 1 h than after 6 h. When the infusion stops the time to a 50% drop in plasma concentration (= V1) will be shorter after the 1-h infusion because the diffusion gradient to V3 is larger.

With a model such as that in Figure 4.3 and data for V1, V2, V3, clearance, and speed of equilibration between the compartments, computerized modeling may be used to predict the relevant plasma concentration in any patient at any time after a given setup for dosing [bolus(es) and/or infusion(s)]. Examples of such modeling are presented in the Stanpump® (http://anesthesia.stanford.edu/pkpd), RUGLOOP® (http://users.skynet.be/fa491447/index.html) and Tivatrainer® (www.eurosiva.org) simulation programs, which are very helpful for understanding intravenous dosing and predicting plasma levels.

The modeling of a fixed iv drug dose depends on the patient's weight, thus weight is always included in such models although often in quite simple ways: doubling the weight means doubling the dose in order to achieve the same plasma concentration. Taking other

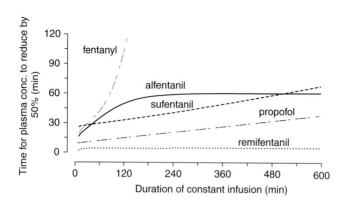

Figure 4.7. Context-sensitive elimination half-life.

patient features into account may increase the precision of prediction, but these are so far often not included because they are difficult to calculate and interpolate into mathematical models of drug pharmacokinetics. Examples are: age, fat or lean (relationship between weight and height), gender, changes in liver or kidney function, etc.

One very important concept for the anesthetist is derived from the pharmacokinetics described above, namely *context-sensitive elimination time*.

Context-sensitive elimination time is the time taken to achieve a predefined reduction of plasma concentration once dosing is stopped. The reduction is a net result of elimination (clearance) plus distribution from the plasma to non-equilibrated tissue. With prolonged exposure, more than 12–24 h, the distribution is negligible (steady-state) and the context-sensitive 50% reduction will be the same as the terminal or steady-state elimination half-life. The term is usually used in conjunction with constant dosing (fixed dose per time), looking for a reduction of 50%, i.e., *the context-sensitive half-time*. Still, it may be used for any kind of dosing schedule and endpoints of 20%, 80%, or any other degree of reduction may be applied. With a carefully titrated and down-adjusted anesthetic for closing a wound it may sometimes be relevant to check for a 20% reduction of analgesic or hypnotic drugs in order to have the patient breathing or awake. Figure 4.7 shows the context-sensitive elimination half-life for propofol and other relevant opioids (see later for individual drug descriptions).

Intravenous drugs: pharmacodynamics

Pharmacodynamics has to do with the following:

a. Timing of onset/offset of effect
b. Strength of effect
c. Type of effect.

Timing of onset/offset of effect

The following steps must take place for a drug to take effect:

- Diffusion out of blood vessels (through the blood–brain barrier)
- Diffusion into extracellular fluid
- Travel to the surface of the effector cell

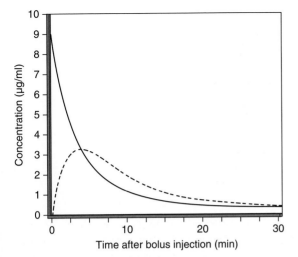

Figure 4.8. Propofol plasma concentration (solid line) after a 2 mg/kg bolus dose in a 70-kg adult. The dotted line is a qualitative estimation of strength of hypnotic effect. The peak effect is about 3–4 min after the start of bolus injection, and depends on: (1) the time taken to travel from the plasma to the CNS and (2) the reducing concentration gradient as the drug is distributed.

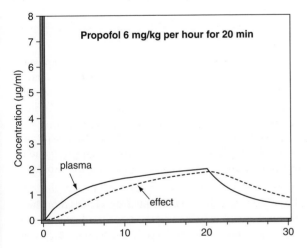

Figure 4.9. Propofol plasma concentration (solid line) during a 6 mg/kg per hour infusion for 20 min in a 70-kg adult. The dotted line is a qualitative estimation of strength of hypnotic effect. The peak effect is about 20 min after the start of the infusion, and depends on: (1) the delay caused as the drug travels from the plasma to the CNS and (2) the plasma concentration rising throughout the period of infusion without reaching a plateau. (The plateau will be reached after 3–5 times the context-sensitive $T\frac{1}{2}$, in this case at about 30–40 min.)

- Bind to a receptor or cell surface or intracellular structure
- Exert biologic effect.

The biologic effect may be fast, such as opening an ion channel; slower, such as activating protein synthesis [e.g., nonsteroidal anti-inflammatory drugs (NSAIDS)]; or slower still, such as activating deoxyribonucleic acid (DNA) and protein synthesis (e.g., corticosteroids). As drugs differ both in their mechanism of biologic effect and in the time taken to get from the plasma to their effect site, they vary in time to onset. This difference may be expressed by a constant, k_{eO}, where a high constant means a rapid onset, or by $T_{1/2}\ k_{eO}$, which is the time taken for 50% equilibration from plasma to effect site. Both these terms are theoretical constructs based on the assumption of a stable plasma concentration, whereas the time to peak effect after a bolus dose is the result of both effect delay and the concentration gradient between the plasma and the brain, which reduces as the drug is distributed (Figure 4.8). With infusion only, the time to peak effect will be prolonged, but this is due rather more to the slow increase in plasma concentration than the delay as the drug travels from the plasma to the effect site (Figure 4.9).

Table 4.1. Delay (min) from drug administration to plasma to onset of effect

	T½ for equilibration between plasma and effect site ($T_{\frac{1}{2}}k_{eO}$) (min)	Time to maximal effect after a bolus dose (min)
Barbiturates (thiopentone)	1.2	1.0–2.0
Propofol	2.6	1.5–3.5
Midazolam	5.6	5–7
Diazepam	2	1–3
Opioids:		
– Remifentanil	1.2	1–2
– Alfentanil	1.1	1.5–3
– Fentanyl	5.8	4–5
– Morphine	?	10–20
NSAID	?	15–30
Corticosteroid	?	60–120

T½ k_{eO} values and time to peak effect for some drugs are given in Table 4.1.

Knowing the time to peak effect after bolus administration is useful in three important contexts:

1. Aim to achieve the maximum effect when the stress is maximal, such as during intubation or the start of surgery.

2. Titrate a drug to the appropriate concentration. Titration involves giving a dose and waiting to observe its full effect. If the full effect is insufficient, a new dose is given and its effect assessed, and so on. The shorter the time to peak effect, the quicker the process of titration.

3. Anticipate the risk of side-effects. For instance, with a slow-acting drug such as morphine, the event of respiratory depression will evolve slowly. Patients become gradually drowsy, then reduce breathing frequency before eventual apnea at the peak effect after 15–20 min. With alfentanil the maximal effect occurs much more rapidly, with sudden apnea occurring perhaps 2 min after a bolus. Thus, with a slow-acting drug you have to observe for longer for safety's sake and titration is relatively slow. A positive aspect though is that you have more time to observe problems emerging and therefore more time to call for help and prepare drugs and equipment as needed.

Strength of effect

Computer programs will usually simulate the time course and changes in relative strength of effect, but not the actual level of clinical effect. For instance, with remifentanil the young and the elderly will have a fairly similar effect site curve, but in the elderly the actual clinical effect may be twice as strong [5]. This is probably due to increased CNS sensitivity to opioids in the elderly and should be taken into account when choosing a dosing level or target plasma or effect-site level in the elderly. It also seems that females need a little more hypnotic agent than males in order to be asleep; again the plasma or effect-site levels of drug may be similar, but the brain sensitivity may differ [6].

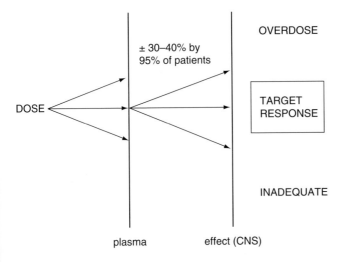

Figure 4.10. A dose (in mg/kg) will result in a spread of plasma concentrations of about ±30–50% around an average, for reasons of pharmacokinetics. Even when a specific plasma target is achieved, there will be a further spread of effect, due to pharmacodynamics.

The strength of effect may be expressed in ways analogous to the MAC for iv drugs: the ED50 or EC50. Effective dose, ED50, is the dose needed in order to bring about desired effect (e.g., sleep, no movement on incision) in 50% of patients; the effective concentration, EC50, is the plasma concentration needed. Generally there is a larger spread of inter-individual effects with iv drugs compared with inhalational drugs; in order to move from the EC50 to EC95 (effective concentration for effect in 95% of patients), the dose needs to be increased by 40–50%; to move from ED50 to ED95, increase dose by 60–80%. The spread of ED will always be larger than the spread of EC, because a dose may result in a variety of plasma concentrations (Figure 4.10). Again, variable effects are seen with all drugs. With EC we anticipate a given plasma concentration and only compensate for variability in sensitivity (Figure 4.10). The inter-individual variability in EC is generally greater for opioids than for hypnotic agents, and we must be prepared for considerable variability in clinical need for opioids compared with other drugs, even in an otherwise normal patient. The range may be fivefold, i.e., the patient with minimal opioid need will require one-fifth of the dose required by a patient with maximal need for the same standardized stimulus.

Type of effect – side-effects

The intravenous anesthetic drugs also have side-effects, the most important and frequently occurring of which are circulatory and respiratory in nature. These different effects arise from a variety of organs and effector cells, and each has a specific time–effect profile and delay (k_{eO}), which differ from those for the basic effects of general anesthesia, hypnosis, and anti-nociception.

Respiratory effects

Opioids cause a dose-dependent reduction in breathing frequency, culminating in apnea. Patients becoming drowsy and a respiratory rate below 8–10 breaths per minute should raise the suspicion of apnea emerging. An inability to maintain a free airway may occur before apnea is present.

Ventilatory depression, being CNS driven, usually follows the analgesic and sedative effects fairly closely. Respiratory depression may be counteracted by stimulation – verbal or (more efficient) tactile and even painful. In a worst case scenario these effects can always be reversed by naloxone, which will also reverse the analgesia abruptly.

The respiratory depression caused by hypnotics is usually regarded as less than that caused by opioids, but it is difficult to sort out equipotency of these two drug classes, as their anesthetic effects are quite different. Respiratory depression is clinically evident as an inability to maintain a free airway and shallow tidal volumes, whereas the spontaneous ventilation frequency may be normal or low. Propofol will always result in apnea with high doses, whereas the benzodiazepines are safer in that very high doses are needed for respiratory arrest, at least in young and fit patients. Full reversal of the effects of benzo-diazepines is also possible with flumazenil.

Circulatory effects

The net circulatory effects are due to a combination of drug effects in the CNS and the periphery (directly in the heart and vessel walls, e.g., vasodilatation), as well as the physio-logic effect of going to sleep with its accompanying reduction in sympathetic nerve tone. A drop in blood pressure (BP) and heart rate during general anesthetic induction is almost always seen (except with ketamine), unless the surgery or other stimulation starts concom-itantly. Although ambulatory patients are slightly hypovolemic (from fasting), they usually tolerate well a short-lasting drop in systolic BP down to the 70–90 mmHg range, as organ blood flow is well maintained and oxygen consumption is low during sleep. Kazama and co-workers have shown that the maximal drop in BP is delayed for 2–3 min when compared with the maximal hypnotic effect of propofol. The BP delay after sleep is 5–6 min in the elderly and the drop is larger, probably due to their having a stiffer myocardium and vessel walls [7].

Intravenous drug interactions: opioids and hypnotics

General anesthesia may be achieved with a very high dose of hypnotic drug alone. A patient with severe benzodiazepine intoxication becomes unconscious and may not react to pain stimuli, thus surgery is possible. Propofol at a dose fivefold higher than that required to induce sleep will achieve the same effect, but this is not practical in terms of drug economy, cardiovascular depression, and speed of recovery. Opioids, in contrast, provide excellent pain relief at high enough doses, but they are not reliable as hypnotics. Although most patients on high-dose opioids will be asleep most of the time, some may be fully awake for periods of time in an unpredictable manner. Thus, general anesthesia with iv drugs only, total intra-venous anesthesia (TIVA), is usually achieved with a combination of opioid and hypnotic drugs, most often propofol.

Opioids reduce the dose of propofol needed for sleep by 20–50% at fairly low doses, such as alfentanil 1–2 mg in an adult, or a remifentanil plasma level of 2.5–5.0 ng/ml. Increasing the opioid dose beyond this does not enable much further dose reduction of propofol for sleep induction.

Thus a minimum dose of propofol of 3–4 mg/kg per hour for maintenance or a target concentration of 1.5–1.8 μg/ml should be used to guarantee sleep, irrespective of high opioid dose.

Propofol reduces the need for opioids for anti-nociception in a dose-dependent manner: anything from a 10–20% reduction with a low sleeping dose (6 mg/kg per hour or a target

Table 4.2.

		Drug			
		Alfentanil	**Fentanyl**	**Sufentanil**	**Remifentanil**
Optimal target with propofol (ng/ml) (EC95)		**130**	**1.6**	**0.2**	**8.0**
Manual dosing for target	1. Bolus (µg/kg) in 30 s	35	3	0.25	2
	2. Infusion (µg/kg per hour)	75 in 30 min	2.5 in 30 min	0.15	22 for 20 min
	3. Infusion thereafter	42	2 for 150 min	same	19
	4. Adjustment	none	to 1.4 after 150 min	none	none
Optimal propofol target (µg/ml) with the opioid (EC95)		**4.4**	**5.4**	**4.5**	**2.8**
Manual dosing for target	1. Bolus (mg/kg) in 30 s	2.8	3.0	2.8	1.5
	2. Infusion (mg/kg per hour) for 40 min	12	15	12	8
	3. Infusion continued for 150 min	10	12	10	6.5
	4. Infusion thereafter	8	11	8	6

(Adapted from Vyuk J et al., *Anesthesiology* 1997:**87**:1549–62):
Recommended combinations of propofol + opioid:
The bold facing indicates the appropriate target concentrations required, whereas the bolus + infusion figure shows the relevant manual dosing for reaching and maintaining that target.

The figures are based on measurements of plasma concentrations of different combinations of alfentanil and propofol during open abdominal surgery, and the optimal combination for the most rapid emergence after 3 h of anesthesia. EC95 figures are the dose combinations needed to keep 95% of the patients completely immobile all the time.

The figures for the other opioids are extrapolated from the alfentanil clinical tests.

Comment: As these figures are based on open laparotomy in curarized patients, in the ambulatory setting we generally give even lower propofol doses (to 1.8–2.2 µg/ml) together with remifentanil unless the patient is paralyzed, but the target level of 2.5–2.8 µg/ml may be appropriate during phases of deep relaxation (i.e., being unable to move).

concentration of 3 µg/ml) to almost 90–100% if the dose is 5–6 times higher (target dose of 15–20 µg/ml).

The practical approach depends on the type of opioid in use as demonstrated by Vuyk and colleagues in their important work on EC50 and EC95 values for propofol + opioid combination in open gastric surgery (Table 4.2).

The main aim with the opioid + propofol combination is to use a high dose of the drug with the shorter context-sensitive elimination half-life. With remifentanil that means having a low and stable concentration of propofol to ensure sleep and then "play" with the opioid dose according to the strength of nociceptive stimulation. This is logical, because the variables during surgery are pain and nociception, whereas the need for the patient to be asleep is invariable. With short-lasting use of fentanyl (or low doses; i.e., 0.1–0.2 mg for procedures less than 30 min, or lower than 0.1 mg/h) the same strategy may be used, namely low-dose propofol to induce sleep. However, if the use of fentanyl is more extensive, a more rapid recovery will be achieved by increasing the propofol dose 100%, which subsequently reduces the need for fentanyl.

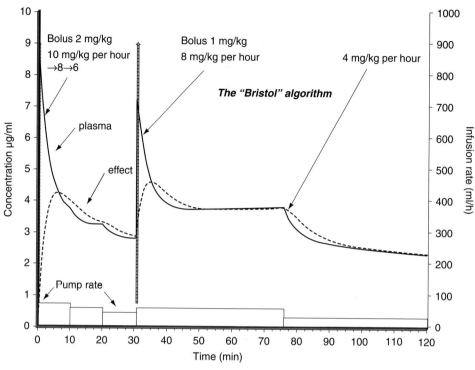

Figure 4.11. Plasma concentration (solid line) and relative strength of hypnotic effect (dotted line) for a manual propofol regime of starting bolus, followed by infusion adjusted at 10 and 20 min. Also shown are an increase in dosing at 30 min and a decrease at 75 min (Marsh kinetic/dynamic model, Tivatrainer®).

As to respiratory depression, opioids are more potent than propofol, and the opioid + propofol combination is synergistic (see "Sedation" in Chapter 5).

Target control infusion [8]

Target control infusion (TCI) is a device to help dose iv drugs with increased precision and less effort. As regards the CNS and clinical effector cells, whether the drug is given by syringe, infusion, or computer is irrelevant; the cells react according to the number of drug molecules present at the effect sites.

With a TCI system you can ensure a rapid onset, a stable effect when needed, a rapid offset or reduction in effect, and less work entailed in dosing and calculation.

The logic of TCI

With a manual scheme for giving propofol, you may achieve a good result and ensure rapid and stable sleep in an adult by adhering to the following recipe: Start with a bolus of 2 mg/kg together with an infusion of 10 mg/kg per hour for 10 min, then adjust the infusion to 8 mg/kg per hour for another 10 min; then adjust to 6 mg/kg per hour which is then maintained for the rest of the case. If this seems to be too much, then adjust the infusion down by 2 mg/kg per minute or if this seems to be too low give another bolus of 0.5 mg/kg and adjust the infusion up with 2 mg/kg per hour. Stop the infusion by the end of the case (Figure 4.11).

This recipe is based on the weight of the patient and simple calculations are made for bolus dose and pump rates. If we call this "Recipe X" we can program a computerized pump to do this automatically. We program the computer with the patient's weight and push the start button: the computer will give the bolus dose and the infusion, and automatically adjusts the rate after 10 and 20 min with no further action by the anesthetist required. If the anesthetist tells the computer to go "up" the computer will deliver a small bolus and adjust the infusion rate. If the anesthetist tells the computer to go "down" the computer pump will stop for a few minutes and then start the infusion at the lower level.

By programming "Recipe X" into the computerized pump we have made a simple TCI plasma system. If we run this program in a series of patients and measure stable plasma propofol concentrations 15 min after the start of the program, we find that the average plasma concentration is about 3 μg/ml (Figure 4.11). Thus we have made a program for our pump to deliver a *plasma target concentration* of 3 μg/ml. If we test the plasma levels 15 min after making the "up" and "down" adjustments, we find concentrations of 4 and 2 μg/ml respectively. Thus, we have made a program to control the pump to increase the target to 4 μg/ml or to reduce the target to 2 μg/ml. By testing different ways of dosing, measuring plasma concentrations (in patients or volunteers), and fitting to mathematical algorithms, we can design programs to dose for any given target in any patient; the only thing we need to tell the computer in the operating theater is the patient's weight and the desired target dose. This is the concept behind the original Marsh *plasma target control infusion* algorithm, which was widely used with propofol-prefilled syringes for pumps programmed with Diprifusor® software (www.eurosiva.org). When testing was done on blood samples, the Marsh algorithm gave quite different plasma levels in different patients (±30–50% around the target) and also tended to give somewhat higher plasma levels than the preset target [9]; despite this, it was still very useful. It provided a stable level and the clinicians soon learnt how to set an appropriate starting target in their patients and how to easily adjust up or down according to clinical need.

A limitation of the Marsh algorithm was that only weight was considered; there was no adjustment for the patient's age or for whether they were obese or slim, simply total weight. This has been the subject of other models, such as Schnider, Schuttler, Paedfusor, etc., in which some of these covariates have been added to calculate dose adjustment.

A major limitation with all models of how to achieve a target plasma level is that they do not take into account the delay in drug equilibration between plasma and CNS. As the anesthetic drug effect is not in plasma, but in the brain, we would prefer a computer pump that delivers a preset concentration to effector sites in the CNS. Thus, we must expand our plasma TCI system into an *effect site TCI system*.

The logic behind such an expansion may be:

We observe that with a plasma target of 3 μg/ml most of our patients will go to sleep, but due to the delay in propofol diffusion from the plasma to the CNS, this will take about 5–10 min, even though the plasma concentration is stable at 3 after 30 s. In order to speed things up, we may "cheat" and tell the pump to start with a target of 6 (Figure 4.11). It still takes 5–10 min to reach this target in the brain, but after 30 s the plasma concentration is 6 and diffusion of drug into the CNS is faster (larger gradient) than with a target of 3. By 2–3 min with a plasma target of 6 we have a CNS concentration of about 3 and the patient goes to sleep. At this point we no longer need to "cheat," but may reduce the plasma target (stop the pump, then restart at a lower rate) to 3. By manipulating the plasma target, we have created an effective algorithm to achieve an effector site (CNS) concentration of 3. Subsequently we can program the computer to do this automatically by the single push of

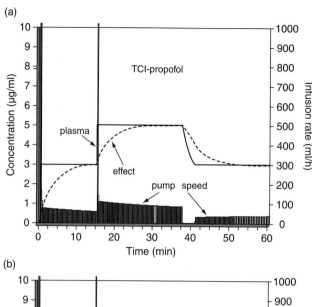

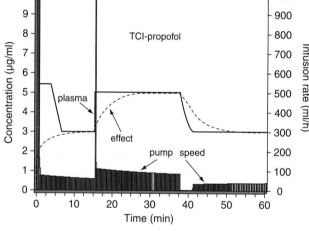

Figure 4.12 (a) Plasma target control infusion, TCI (pump rate indicated by black columns) for a target of 3, then 5, then back to 3. Note that the pump gives a short-lasting bolus injection both at the start and when increasing the dose, and decreases the dose through temporary stoppage. Also note that the pump rate is adjusted far more frequently (= more accurately) than is the case with a manual regimen (as in Figure 4.11). Also note the delay in effect, the patient is probably not asleep until 5–7 min. (b) Same as in Fig 4.12, except for "cheating" with a plasma target of 5.5 μg/min during induction, in order to obtain a more rapid effect (dotted curve); the patient will probably be asleep at 2–3 min.

the button, asking for an effector site target dose of 3 to be delivered. The algorithms for effect site TCI work by overshooting the plasma level to start with or by increasing target levels, and by having prolonged pump stoppages and undershooting plasma levels when we want to reduce the target (Figure. 4.12a).

A problem with effect site modeling is that the delay until an effect is seen is quite variable between individuals, and also somewhat dependent on the rate of bolus/dosing, the dose level (high or low), the patient's cardiovascular status, etc. Also, the delay is hard to measure exactly and the relationship depends on both arterial and venous drug concentration, which vary with changes in dosing. Nevertheless, effect-site modeling is getting better and has proven to be very useful clinically.

Plasma-concentration TCI and effect-site TCI are also being used with remifentanil, and for other opioids, such as alfentanil, fentanyl, and sufentanil.

Different TCI models

Plasma-concentration versus effect-site models

How does one decide between a plasma-concentration and an effect-site TCI model? The general rule is to use the effect-site mode, as this is simpler to use and closer to drug physiology. Nevertheless, one may do quite well with a plasma-concentration TCI, and it should be remembered that the difference in dosing between plasma-concentration TCI and effect-site TCI only occurs during the first 10–15 min after each change (or start) in dosing; under stable conditions they are the same. Using plasma-concentration TCI one should remember to overshoot the target at the start and when a rapid increase in effect is required. When using effect-site TCI one should remember that a higher bolus dose is given every time the dose is increased, and that this may exert a stronger effect on breathing and hemodynamics.

Remifentanil

For remifentanil there is only one model in major clinical use, the Minto model for both plasma-concentration and effect-site modes [10]. The Minto model hits the target well on average, but a ±30–50% deviation may be observed between individual patients [9]. For plasma-concentration modeling, the patient's weight versus height ratio and age are both taken into account. When used in the effect-site mode, it will only deliver a drug "concentration" in the CNS and will not be adjusted for the patient's sensitivity to drug concentration (dynamics). For instance, with no stimulation and effect-site infusion of 2 ng/ml, a 20-year-old patient may be breathing and awake, whereas an 80-year-old patient probably will be asleep and have apnea. This is because opioid sensitivity in the elderly is about twice that seen in younger patients. The drug sensitivity is not built into the models, only drug concentration.

Propofol

With propofol there have been a number of groups who have made TCI models based on their measurements of plasma and effect delay in their series of patients or volunteers. Such measurements are not exact and the results will also differ between individuals. For this reason, it is no surprise that different authors have developed different models. The basic differences between models are in their estimation of the size of V1 (see Figure 4.4) and the delay of effect. In essence, if a model concludes that V1 is large, then the initial dosing (in mg/kg) should be large, and if the delay is long (low k_{eO}, long $T_{1/2}\ k_{eO}$) the initial dose (overshoot) in effect-site mode should be large. These differences are evident in the first 15 min of a case, after which time the models will behave fairly similarly.

Also, it should be noted that some models compensate for the weight/height ratio and/or age, whereas others only compensate for total weight. The common models do not compensate for differences in propofol sensitivity, as may be decreased in children and slightly in females. For more detailed discussion on models one is referred elsewhere [8], but some general statements can be made:

- Marsh plasma-concentration TCI [11]: generally delivers somewhat more than predicted, especially at the start (high V1).
- Marsh effect – old: this model has a long delay in effect and will tend to overdose initially compared with measurements in patients.
- Marsh effect – new [12]: this model has a very short delay in effect, which will compensate somewhat for the overdosing in the plasma part of the algorithm.

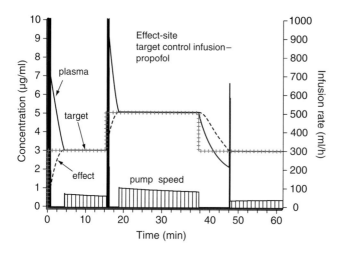

Figure 4.13. Effect-site TCI for propofol. The pump is programmed to deliver an effect-site level of 3, then 5, then 3 again. Note the differences from Figure 4.12 and plasma-concentration TCI. At the start and when increasing the dose there will be a plasma "overshoot" created by a faster bolus infusion, followed by cessation for proper equilibration with the effect site. To decrease the effect-site concentration, the pump is stopped and the plasma concentration allowed to fall below the new target level, after which a small bolus is given to "catch up" with the effect curve and maintain the new level stable.

The clinical impression is that the delay is too short in this model and a 100% overshoot in target for 1–2 min at the start of a case will work better in terms of sending the patient to sleep within 2–3 min.

- Schnider – plasma-concentration TCI: the Schnider model [13] was not actually developed for the plasma-concentration mode, and will underdose the patients initially (low V1). If used, the starting target should be 50–100% higher than with the Marsh model in order to deliver the same dose (mg/kg).

- Schnider – effect-site mode: this has an intermediate delay in effect, which will compensate somewhat for the underdosing in plasma-concentration mode. It also compensates to some extent for thin/fat patients and the elderly. The target levels need to be a little higher (+10–20%) than those in the Marsh models. In the very obese, the formula for weight correction will be wrong, and the model should not be used for patients heavier than 100–120 kg total weight without further adjustment.

- Kataria/Paedfusor: none of the above models compensates for the patient being a child. Children have a higher V1 and a higher clearance in relation to weight than adults. Both these models for children will compensate for these features, resulting in a higher and more appropriate dose for a given target, both for starting and maintenance doses in children.

Anesthesiologic drugs; some practical comments

This section does not provide thorough, systematic information about the indications, contraindications, and dosing for drugs as provided in a drug manual or a textbook of pharmacology. The idea is to provide some personal, practical clinical comments.

Inhalational agents

These should only be used where an appropriate scavenger system is present. However, it may be acceptable to use them occasionally for a very short period (5–10 min) in a well-ventilated room without a scavenger if there is a good indication for their use. Such indications are a child not accepting iv induction, sudden bronchospasm, or sudden arousal of a patient during a case. For sudden bronchospasm I try 2–4% sevoflurane for 5–10 min, then tapering down while checking airway resistance (auscultation and/ or pressure on the ventilator). For sudden arousal, it is always wise to give a bolus of propofol or opioid, but the most rapid way of getting control is to turn the sevoflurane vaporizer to 8% and give four to five rapid breaths, then tapering down and eventually giving iv drugs.

In situations where there is a need for a rapid inhalational effect, I will use a high fresh gas flow of oxygen or oxygen-air at 6–8 l/min.

In general, it may be wise to use a high fresh gas flow (6 l/min in adults) for 10–15 min during induction and at the end of the case, otherwise reducing to a fresh gas flow of 1.5–2 l/min for reasons of economy and improved humidity regulation. With low flow the use of an end-tidal gas monitor is mandatory; with high flow one may do without, although monitoring is still recommended.

Sevoflurane is the routinely used potent gas, because of its low irritation and pungency. I will avoid using it for maintenance in prolonged cases (tissue accumulation) and also as the only drug for maintenance and emergence when anesthetizing children.

Desflurane is not suited for induction or when a strong effect is needed suddenly, but it is well suited for maintenance and also for emergence when anesthetizing children, having as it does a lower rate of emergence delirium compared with sevoflurane. Desflurane is well suited for optimal emergence (faster than propofol) after prolonged procedures, such as eye surgery and dental surgery. In such cases the surgeon should be encouraged to use optimal techniques of local anesthesia for anti-nociception, and a desflurane component of 2–3% may be used solely to ensure reliable sleep. In fat patients the benefit of a rapid, clearheaded recovery after desflurane is evident when compared with sevoflurane or propofol after 1–2 h of anesthesia, and more so for prolonged procedures. One study also suggests that desflurane may result in less "sleepiness" in the days following cholecystectomy, compared with propofol maintenance [14].

Isoflurane is a well-documented and cheaper alternative to sevoflurane and desflurane. The recovery is slower, but with careful down titration towards the end of the procedure, emergence may be rapid [15].

Nitrous oxide is less potent and also associated with nausea and vomiting, as with other inhalational agents. Controversy still surrounds the potential of nitrous oxide to cause postoperative nausea and vomiting (PONV). Some dental patients are certainly nauseated by nitrous oxide alone and the risk increases in patients with a high baseline PONV risk. However, there are also some good, large studies showing no impact of nitrous oxide if the risk of PONV otherwise is low during a general anesthetic case. My conclusion is to avoid nitrous oxide in people with a very high risk of PONV, but otherwise I like to use it routinely when it is available and there is a proper scavenger system in place. Its advantages are its rapid on–off effect, the best of all our drugs; its minor influence on ventilation and circulation; and the resulting 20–40% reduction in dose of other drugs which may be achieved by simultaneous administration of nitrous oxide. When given together with a totally iv technique, the propofol dose may be reduced by one-third. Also, there is benefit in having nitrous oxide running if anything goes wrong with the infusion, iv cannula, pump, etc.

Intravenous hypnotics

Barbiturates

Although rarely used in modern ambulatory anesthesia, they are a low-cost alternative to propofol.

a. Thiopentone

This should only be used for induction or for one to two repeated doses per case for a maximum of 10–15 min, as its elimination is very slow. The onset of effect is a little faster than with propofol, but this is not important in elective cases.

b. Methohexital

This is fairly rapidly cleared and eliminated and may be used as a "poor man's infusion" for TIVA. It is tricky to evaluate and titrate as the patients may have involuntary movements and quite strong aching during induction as well as hiccups [16,17].

Diazepam

This has a slow elimination rate and active metabolites, but seems to be a little less hypnotic and thus more anxiolytic than midazolam. It is a good choice for premedication, 5–10 mg orally, especially if the patient needs an anxiolytic for more than 1–2 h ahead of surgery. It is also a good choice in the recovery unit when a patient feels restless or anxious (2.5 mg iv, repeated).

Midazolam

This is hypnotic, anxiolytic, and amnesic. Midazolam is short acting with no active metabolites, and has a clear drop in effect after 2 h. It is well suited for premedication when there is less than 2 h until the start of anesthesia, either orally 5–7.5 mg or iv 2.5–5.0 mg. The habit of using midazolam before or as a part of the iv induction of anesthesia is not so well founded; a minor dose of propofol will have a similar effect and there is no rationale for reducing the propofol dose with midazolam, as the latter has a potentially slower recovery.

Propofol

Propofol is the "gold standard" hypnotic for ambulatory anesthesia. In low doses it will have anxiolytic, amnesic, and anti-emetic properties, and is also the drug of choice for sedation. Propofol has rapid metabolism and rapid recovery, although emergence may take a few minutes more than with sevoflurane or desflurane, unless the propofol dose is tapered carefully down by the end of anesthesia. However, recovery is pleasant, the patient often feeling slightly euphoric, it has an anti-emetic effect and a low incidence of shivering.

Propofol may ache in thin veins at the start of dosing; the aching may be avoided by using a large vein, for instance in the elbow. Propofol in medium-chain triglyceride solute causes less of an ache, as does the 5 mg/ml solution (e.g., children) compared with 10 mg/ml. Further tricks to reduce aching may be to inject lidocaine 10 mg/ml, 2–3 ml first (best with a tourniquet for 1–2 min, but it also works without a tourniquet), to give an iv opioid first, or to mix lidocaine 10 mg/ml, 1 ml into 10 ml propofol shortly before injection. Such lidocaine-mixed propofol should be used within a few hours, otherwise the lipid emulsion will become unstable. It has also been shown that using a local anesthesia pad (e.g., EMLA®) may further reduce the incidence of aching from propofol in the same area. Although propofol contains soya oil, this is treated and free of antigens, thus hardly any cases of true propofol allergy are reported in the literature.

In a situation that has been stable since the previous dose adjustment (more than 15–20 min), a propofol infusion of 6 mg/kg per hour will correspond to a target (plasma or effect site) of about 2.5 µg/ml.

Dexmedetomidine [18]

Dexmedetomidine is a highly selective α2 adrenoreceptor agonist with both sedative and analgesic effects with minimal respiratory depression. Dexmedetomidine induces a physiologic-like sleep (i.e., deep non-rapid-eye-movement (REM) sleep), in that patients may be very clearheaded immediately after emergence from this drug [19].

Dexmedetomidine may induce hypotension, bradycardia, and a dry mouth, and has an anti-shivering effect. It is still not approved in Europe, but shows potential as a valuable drug in terms of sedation and opioid-sparing effects perioperatively. Dexmedetomidine has been used successfully for sedation in children, whereas its role in adult sedation requires better elucidation. Although theoretically attractive, it seems to have a slower onset and offset than propofol, meaning that it may not be ideal in the ambulatory setting. Nevertheless, as an adjunct it may play an important role in the future.

Opioids

Fentanyl

May result in prolonged emergence and thus more PONV when used in high doses, but may still be useful for short procedures of 15–30 min if the total dose is less than 0.2 mg in the adult. Used together with remifentanil it is our routine to give 0.05–0.1 mg (adults, children 1 µg/kg) by the end of remifentanil-based anesthesia, in order to avoid having a patient wake up with no opioid effect and strong pain. Fentanyl is our favorite opioid for postoperative pain relief within the first 1–2 h, as it works fairly rapidly in 0.05-mg increments (0.5 µg/kg in children) with a weaning of effect and side-effects after 20–30 min. There is no rationale for using fentanyl together with remifentanil at induction or for maintenance during a case; a better choice is to dose only remifentanil as needed [20].

Alfentanil

A simple, ampoule-ready, alternative to remifentanil for short cases and for handling strong and short-lasting nociceptive stimulation. Alfentanil has a peak effect at 1–2 min and declines after 10–15 min. A dose of 1.5–2.0 mg may work very well for procedures of 10–20 min in adults, perhaps with 0.5 mg supplemented as needed (in children 25 mg/kg for 5–10 min of surgery, supplemented with 10 mg/kg as needed). As alfentanil works fast, it may induce a stiff chest if dosed beyond 2–3 mg in an adult who has not received hypnotics first [21].

Remifentanil

In many ways remifentanil is the ideal opioid for ambulatory care; its rapid peak of effect occurs within 1–2 min and it never takes longer than 3–4 min for 50% recovery following cessation of administration even after very prolonged dosing [22]. Remifentanil has to be prepared from a powder, and will be given by an infusion pump. With an infusion of less than 0.1 µg/kg per minute there is a fair chance of maintaining spontaneous breathing, but for surgery usually a dose of 0.2–0.5 µg/kg is needed. It may also be given in bolus doses, 0.5–1 µg/kg, repeated every 5 min. In order to tolerate laryngeal mask insertion, a rule of thumb is to ensure a dose of 2 µg/kg given over 2–3 min, whereas for intubation without curare a dose of 3–4 µg/kg is needed. One should be aware of the risk of a stiff chest with any dose of more than 1 µg/kg given rapidly (within 1 min) to a patient, the elderly being more prone to this complication. However, a stiff chest only occurs if no hypnotic drug is given first, thus with an induction dose of propofol (or midazolam) given beforehand, high and rapid doses of remifentanil will be well tolerated.

Concern has been raised over the hyperalgesic effects of remifentanil, seen experimentally after only 30 min of infusion, and clinically after more than 2–3 hours of infusions of more than 0.3 µg/kg per minute. Clinically, these patients have a lowered pain threshold post-operatively for some hours, with increased need for opioid and non-opioid analgesics. It is disputed whether remifentanil is worse than other opioids in this respect, or whether it is just more easily seen as the remifentanil analgesic effect is so short-lasting and the peroperative dosing is more generous than with other opioids. It is our impression that this hyperalgesia is not a problem if the remifentanil dose is kept at or below 0.3 µg/kg per minute; but it may be seen if the dose is above the range of 0.3–0.4 µg/kg for more than 1–2 h [20]. Experimental data suggest that in such cases hyperalgesia may be prevented effectively with a low-dose (1–2 µg/kg per minute) infusion of ketamine [23], and probably also partially by NSAIDs or cyclooxygenase inhibitors given preoperatively or potent inhalational anesthesia supplemented peroperatively.

In a stable situation (more than 5–10 min after the last adjustment) a remifentanil infusion of 0.1 µg/kg per minute will correspond to a target (plasma or effect-site concentration) of about 2.5 ng/ml.

Sufentanil

Sufentanil behaves fairly similarly to fentanyl for limited use, as in ambulatory care, but has a slightly slower onset and no specific features for use in this setting.

Oxycodone

Oxycodone is the opioid with the highest and most predictable bioavailability (70–80%) after oral dosing. It is well suited for extra analgesia after discharge for 1–3 days in patients who have pain problems in spite of optimal non-opioid medication. It may be used in sustained release tablet form twice a day; usually 10 mg will do but some cases may need 20 mg. This may be supplemented by ordinary 5-mg tablets, taken as needed, but always wait for 1 hour before taking more. Oxycodone may also be used intravenously, and is probably slightly more (+25–50%) potent than morphine. Some studies suggest that oxycodone has a little less-sedative profile compared with morphine and may be better for visceral postoperative pain [24].

Codeine

Codeine has a lower bioavailability than oxycodone (50–60%) and works through degradation by cytochrome P-450 type 2D6 to morphine in the body. Some 5–10% of Caucasians have a failure of this enzyme and codeine will have almost no clinical effect for them. In contrast, 0.5–1% of Caucasians may be extensive metabolizers and for them codeine has a very strong effect. For these reasons the effect of codeine unpredictable and slow.

Codeine is still very popular as an oral opioid, often in conjunction with paracetamol (acetaminophen). With combination preparations care should be taken to give the patient the proper paracetamol dose, that is with a low dose of codeine + paracetamol combination, some paracetamol tablets should be added to the regime. When giving the combination of paracetamol and codeine to supplement an optimal dose of paracetamol alone, care should be taken to avoid overdosing of paracetamol.

Non-opioid analgesics

These are dealt with in more detail in Chapter 6. In order to avoid opioid-induced side-effects postoperatively it is important to provide optimal non-opioid analgesia before transfer to the postanesthesia care unit (PACU). The cornerstones are paracetamol, NSAIDs or cyclo-oxygenase inhibitors, glucocorticoids, and local anesthesia applied directly to the wounds.

Neuromuscular blockers and reversal agents

In modern anesthesia and ambulatory care in particular, the use of neuromuscular blockers has declined, and they should only be used when specifically indicated. Use of muscle relaxants necessitates extra drugs, which has implications for cost and potential side-effects. Very often reversal and anticholinergic agents are also needed and there is a rare risk of serious awareness, which is not seen in non-curarized patients who always move if they are in discomfort [25].

Indications for neuromuscular blockers:

a. The surgeon needs strong relaxation of patient muscle in order to access anatomic structures. This may be the case with laparotomies, thoracotomies, and major joint surgery. In ambulatory cases this need is rare, but may be indicated in some cases of laparoscopy, e.g., in the obese or patients with many adhesions. When needed the dose can be low, about 50% of intubating dose, i.e., two to three twitches on TOF guard (train-of-four) neuromuscular monitor.

b. The surgeon sometimes needs the patient to lie completely still; even a small movement may ruin the result. This may be the case for some ambulatory procedures, such as microsurgery on vessels, the middle ear, or the eye. In these cases a TOF guard should always be used and one should maintain a dosing that ensures either one or no twitches during the critical periods and be prepared to use reversal agents to end the case.

c. The anesthesiologist needs to do a rapid sequence induction in the acutely ill or non-fasting patient in order to secure the airway rapidly. This indication is virtually nonexistent in ambulatory care; if there is a suspicion of non-fasting status, the patient's surgery should be postponed until an empty stomach is assured.

d. The anesthesiologist needs a neuromuscular blocker for routine elective intubation. Again, the use of an endotracheal tube should be fairly infrequent in ambulatory care, but there are exceptions: oral surgery, dental surgery, tonsillectomies, and obese patients for laparoscopies. In fairly healthy patients the intubation may be done with a combination of remifentanil and propofol (see Chapter 7). Although minor mucous membrane damage has been reported, and coughing sometimes occurs, there are very few reports of serious problems or prolonged disability due to this approach [26–28].

e. The anesthesiologist needs a neuromuscular blocker for gentle induction with intubation in the elderly or otherwise fragile patient. This indication is also advantageous in that the use of high-dose remifentanil + propofol in elderly patients may result in an unpredictable drop in blood pressure; thus, concomitant use of neuromuscular blocker allows the dosing of anesthetics to be kept lower and the circulation more stable during intubation.

f. The anesthesiologist needs to use neuromuscular blockers to resolve a stiff chest (high-dose remifentanil or alfentanil in a nonsedated patient) or laryngospasm (in a child during induction or emergence, or patient with sudden, strong surgical peroperative stimulation).

Suxamethonium

Suxamethonium is a cheap, fast-onset, and short-acting drug with no need or effect of reversal.

Use in ambulatory patients may result in muscular pain for 1–2 days due to the contractions induced to begin with. In many countries it remains the anesthesiologic drug with highest incidence of anaphylactic reactions. About 1 in 4000 patients may also have an unexpected metabolic deficiency that calls for antiserum or ventilation and sedation for 3–4 h until the block resolves.

Mivacurium

A fairly short-acting (20–40 min) nondepolarizing drug that does not require reversal routinely, and that has organ-independent metabolism. Cases of degradation enzyme deficiencies occur, as with suxamethonium. Fairly slow onset, over 3–4 min.

Vecuronium, cisatracurium

Well-established, safe alternatives for nondepolarizing block, fairly slow onset (3–4 min) and offset, should always be used in conjunction with TOF guard monitoring. These drugs usually have to be combined with neostigmine + glycopyrrolate reversal, which should only be attempted when more than two to three twitches register on the TOF guard.

Rocuronium

Acts faster than other nondepolarizing agents, especially when dosed high; onset down to 1 min, comparable with suxamethonium. The downside of such dosing is its very prolonged effect, for hours, which may be counteracted efficiently at any time with sugammadex. Discussion about the more frequent anaphylaxis seen with this drug in some countries (France and Norway) is not fully conclusive; the incidence still seems to be low and comparable with that of alternatives [29].

Neuromuscular reversal

Reports of serious clinical problems of residual neuromuscular block during recovery are rare, but an increased incidence of pulmonary complications in the elderly has been demonstrated with poor reversal of block [30]. Newer studies suggest that a TOF ratio of anything less than 0.9 (i.e., fourth twitch strength is 90% that of the first twitch) may interfere with normal swallowing and thus lead to risk of aspiration [31].

Neostigmine + glycopyrrolate combination

Even with a partial block, i.e., one or two twitches on the TOF guard, it takes 10–20 min for full reversal of block in some patients [32]. The dose should be 50–70 μg/kg in order to be adequate. With this dose the risk of nausea and vomiting is increased, almost doubled in one study [33], and also other side-effects may be seen such as bronchial constriction or defecation.

Sugammadex

Sugammadex is a very elegant and rapid reversal agent for rocuronium and vecuronium only. Reversal within 1–2 min may be achieved at any level of muscle relaxation. This may be relevant to microsurgery when the surgeon finishes suddenly or even in the case of difficult intubation, when a high dose of rocuronium may be reversed by a high dose of sugammadex. Other indications are poor pulmonary function and the very obese patient, for whom complete and rapid reversal may reduce the risk of complications. The main problem is the cost, about 100 euro for a standard dose of 2 mg/kg and two to four times greater if a high dose is used for profound block. Nevertheless, unpublished work suggests that a small dose of 0.5 mg/kg may be sufficient for an average block and may even be combined with neostigmine for dose reduction.

Ketamine [23]

Ketamine is an N-methyl-D-aspartate (NMDA) receptor blocker with dose-dependent analgesic, hypnotic, and some muscle relaxant effects. Spontaneous breathing is maintained. In contrast with other general anesthetics, ketamine stimulates the sympathetic nervous system to maintain blood pressure and heart rate when the patient falls asleep. For this reason ketamine is often the routine induction drug of choice in hypovolemic or severely bleeding patients. Because of its simplicity of use, ketamine is also much used in field situations or in places with limited resources. A problem with ketamine is the significant occurrence of bad dreams and hallucinations during emergence, which may be partly, but not completely, counteracted by a concomitant benzodiazepine.

As ambulatory anesthesia is particularly concerned with achieving rapid and uneventful recovery and is rarely undertaken in hypovolemic patients or field situations, ketamine traditionally has a very limited role in ambulatory care. Nevertheless, two recent issues have challenged this view: one is the claim that ketamine is an ideal sedative when given in conjunction with propofol and the other is research on the role of the NMDA receptor in hyperalgesia and chronic pain.

a.   Although ketamine is traditionally associated with slow emergence and some incidence of unpleasant hallucinations, even when given in moderate doses for sedation [34], Friedberg et al. have repeatedly reported a high success rate for ketamine-induced sedation during plastic surgery under local anesthesia. Propofol, increasingly supplemented with ketamine for light or profound sedation during spontaneous ventilation, gave no hallucinations and virtually no postoperative nausea and vomiting (PONV) [35,36]. Recent publications in the ambulatory setting partly support this conclusion [37]. However, Aouad et al. reported increased agitation [38,39], Goel et al. reported delayed recovery [40], and a review by Slavik and Zed concluded that there are no specific benefits of this technique [41].

For this discussion it should be noted that this technique is mainly reported when carried out with sedation for plastic surgery and thorough local anesthesia infiltration to provide basic analgesia. The propofol doses have been fairly generous and the ketamine doses fairly low. To date, one randomized, double-blind study on the benefit of this technique has demonstrated improved cardiovascular stability when a single dose of ketamine (0.3 mg/kg) is compared with fentanyl (1.5 µg/kg) during propofol sedation [37].

b. Recent interest has also been shown in low-dose ketamine infusion for the reduction of postoperative pain and hyperalgesia [42,43]. As NMDA activation appears to be involved in the development of opioid-induced hyperalgesia, low-dose ketamine infusion has proven efficacious at blunting hyperalgesia [43]. For this antihyperalgesic effect a continuous infusion (1–2 µg/kg per minute, throughout the whole perioperative period including 1–2 days postoperatively) seems to be best, although the clinical relevance of hyperalgesia in ambulatory anesthesia is not well documented. However, ketamine also has direct analgesic effects, given as a single bolus dose (0.15–0.5 mg/kg) or as a peroperative infusion. The meta-analyses of both Bell et al. [44] and Elia [45] concluded on a postoperative opioid-sparing effect and no significant side-effects from using a ketamine adjunct. One study of 0.15 mg/kg given preoperatively also suggests a pre-emptive effect after gynecologic surgery, as the group receiving the preoperative dose had better analgesia than the postoperative dosing group [46]. Nevertheless, while some studies are positive [47], others do not find any effect apart from short-lasting analgesia together with increased postoperative sedation [48].

In conclusion, ketamine may be a promising alternative to low-dose opioids as an adjunct to propofol sedation with safe, spontaneous breathing. However, more studies are needed on both this issue and the clinical benefits of ketamine for analgesia after ambulatory surgery.

Anti-emetics

These are dealt with in Chapter 6; in the section on postoperative nausea and vomiting (PONV).

Acute drugs – rescue situations

These drugs should be immediately available (i.e., ampoules on your table together with syringe and needle) for all cases of anesthetic care:

- *Atropine*: for bradycardia, usually I accept a heart rate down to 40 beats per minute if the patient is stable, has an adequate BP, and sinus rhythm. If needed, start at 0.5 mg iv (adult).
- *Ephedrine*: versatile vasoconstrictive drug for hypotension; start with 5–10 mg iv. Alternatively phenylephrine (0.5–1 µg/kg) or in more resistant cases adrenaline (0.1 mg). In the healthy adult with a running crystalloid infusion I usually accept a short-lasting (few minutes) fall in systolic BP to 80 mmHg without intervention; placing the patient head down may be an alternative.
- *Beta-blocker*: an iv beta-blocker (esmolol or metoprolol) may be needed for tachycardia, arrhythmia, or hypertension. Usually start with 2–3 mg metoprolol, then titrate 1 mg every 3–4 min while watching the ECG continuously. Also, one group reported that an experimental technique of using esmolol infusion (5–15 µg/kg per minute) obviated the need for opioids and improved postoperative function and analgesia [49].
- *Adrenaline*: for anaphylactic reactions; 0.2–0.3 mg iv, then titrated against effect on anaphylaxis with low BP and/or severe bronchospasm.
- *Antagonists*: opioid (naloxone 0.1 mg titrated) and benzodiazepine (flumazenil 0.1 mg titrated) antagonists should always be readily available.

- *Intralipid*: a small bottle should be available when using bupivacaine for local anesthesia, as intralipid is an effective scavenger of bupivacaine in cases of toxicity.
- *Equipment for emergency airway handling and induction of general anesthesia*: this will include laryngoscopes, stylets, oral airway, LMA (basic and fast-track), suxamethonium, propofol, fluids, self-inflating bag, masks, etc.

References

1. Einarsson SG, Cerne A, Bengtsson A, et al. Respiration during emergence from anaesthesia with desflurane/N$_2$O vs. desflurane/air for gynaecological laparoscopy. *Acta Anaesthesiol Scand* 1998;**42**:1192–8.

2. Katoh T, Ikeda K. The effects of fentanyl on sevoflurane requirements for loss of consciousness and skin incision. *Anesthesiology* 1998;**88**:18–24.

3. Albertin A, Dedola E, Bergonzi PC, et al. The effect of adding two target-controlled concentrations (1–3 ng ml^{-1}) of remifentanil on MAC BAR of desflurane. *Eur J Anaesthesiol* 2006;**23**:510–16.

4. Inagaki Y, Sumikawa K, Yoshiya I. Anesthetic interaction between midazolam and halothane in humans. *Anesth Analg* 1993;**76**:613–17.

5. Minto CF, Schnider TW, Egan TD, et al. Influence of age and gender on the pharmacokinetics and pharmacodynamics of remifentanil. I. Model development. *Anesthesiology* 1997;**86**:10–23.

6. Hoymork SC, Raeder J. Why do women wake up faster than men from propofol anaesthesia? *Br J Anaesth* 2005;**95**:627–33.

7. Kazama T, Ikeda K, Morita K, et al. Comparison of the effect-site k(eO)s of propofol for blood pressure and EEG bispectral index in elderly and younger patients. *Anesthesiology* 1999;**90**:1517–27.

8. Absalom AR, Struys MRF. *An overview of TCI and TIVA*, Ghent: Academia Press, 2005.

9. Hoymork SC, Raeder J, Grimsmo B, Steen PA. Bispectral index, predicted and measured drug levels of target-controlled infusions of remifentanil and propofol during laparoscopic cholecystectomy and emergence. *Acta Anaesthesiol Scand* 2000;**44**:1138–44.

10. Minto CF, Schnider TW, Shafer SL. Pharmacokinetics and pharmacodynamics of remifentanil. II. Model application. *Anesthesiology* 1997;**86**:24–33.

11. Kenny GN, White M. A portable computerised infusion system for propofol. *Anaesthesia* 1990;**45**:692–3.

12. Vereecke HE, Vasquez PM, Jensen EW, et al. New composite index based on midlatency auditory evoked potential and electroencephalographic parameters to optimize correlation with propofol effect site concentration: comparison with bispectral index and solitary used fast extracting auditory evoked potential index. *Anesthesiology* 2005;**103**:500–7.

13. Minto CF, Schnider TW, Gregg KM, et al. Using the time of maximum effect site concentration to combine pharmacokinetics and pharmacodynamics. *Anesthesiology* 2003;**99**:324–33.

14. Mjaland O, Raeder J, Aasboe V, et al. Outpatient laparoscopic cholecystectomy. *Br J Surg* 1997;**84**:958–61.

15. Seitsonen ER, Yli-Hankala AM, Korttila KT. Similar recovery from bispectral index-titrated isoflurane and sevoflurane anesthesia after outpatient gynecological surgery. *J Clin Anesth* 2006;**18**:272–9.

16. Raeder JC, Misvaer G. Comparison of propofol induction with thiopentone or methohexitone in short outpatient general anaesthesia. *Acta Anaesthesiol Scand* 1988;**32**:607–13.

17. Lee JS, Gonzalez ML, Chuang SK, Perrott DH. Comparison of methohexital and propofol use in ambulatory procedures in oral and maxillofacial surgery. *J Oral Maxillofac Surg* 2008;**66**:1996–2003.

18. Carollo DS, Nossaman BD, Ramadhyani U. Dexmedetomidine: a review of clinical applications. *Curr Opin Anaesthesiol* 2008;**21**:457–61.

19. Sanders RD, Maze M. Alpha2-adrenoceptor agonists. *Curr Opin Investig Drugs* 2007;**8**:25–33.

20. Lenz H, Raeder J, Hoymork SC. Administration of fentanyl before remifentanil-based anaesthesia has no influence on post-operative pain or analgesic consumption. *Acta Anaesthesiol Scand* 2008;**52**:149–54.

21. Raeder JC, Hole A. Alfentanil anaesthesia in gall-bladder surgery. *Acta Anaesthesiol Scand* 1986;**30**:35–40.

22. Raeder J. Remifentanil, a new age in anaesthesia? In: Vuyk J, Engbers F, Groen-Mulder S, eds. *On the Study and Practice of Intravenous Anaesthesia*, Dordrecht: Kluwer Academic, 2000: 249–60.

23. Raeder JC, Stenseth LB. Ketamine: a new look at an old drug. *Curr Opin Anaesthesiol* 2000;**13**:463–8.

24. Lenz H, Sandvik L, Qvigstad E, et al. A comparison of intravenous oxycodone and intravenous morphine in patient-controlled postoperative analgesia after laparoscopic hysterectomy. *Anesth Analg* 2009;**109**:1279–83.

25. Sandin RH, Enlund G, Samuelsson P, Lennmarken C. Awareness during anaesthesia: a prospective case study. *Lancet* 2000;**355**:707–11.

26. McNeil IA, Culbert B, Russell I. Comparison of intubating conditions following propofol and succinylcholine with propofol and remifentanil 2 µg kg^{-1} or 4 µg kg^{-1}. *Br J Anaesth* 2000;**85**:623–5.

27. Mencke T, Echternach M, Kleinschmidt S, et al. Laryngeal morbidity and quality of tracheal intubation: a randomized controlled trial. *Anesthesiology* 2003;**98**:1049–56.

28. Stevens JB, Wheatley L. Tracheal intubation in ambulatory surgery patients: using remifentanil and propofol without muscle relaxants. *Anesth Analg* 1998;**86**:45–9.

29. Harboe T, Guttormsen AB, Irgens A, et al. Anaphylaxis during anesthesia in Norway: a 6-year single-center follow-up study. *Anesthesiology* 2005;**102**:897–903.

30. Berg H, Roed J, Viby-Mogensen J, et al. Residual neuromuscular block is a risk factor for postoperative pulmonary complications. A prospective, randomised, and blinded study of postoperative pulmonary complications after atracurium, vecuronium and pancuronium. *Acta Anaesthesiol Scand* 1997;**41**:1095–103.

31. Eriksson LI, Sundman E, Olsson R, et al. Functional assessment of the pharynx at rest and during swallowing in partially paralyzed humans: simultaneous videomanometry and mechanomyography of awake human volunteers. *Anesthesiology* 1997;**87**:1035–43.

32. Kirkegaard H, Heier T, Caldwell JE. Efficacy of tactile-guided reversal from cisatracurium-induced neuromuscular block. *Anesthesiology* 2002;**96**:45–50.

33. Lovstad RZ, Thagaard KS, Berner NS, Raeder JC. Neostigmine 50 µg kg^{-1} with glycopyrrolate increases postoperative nausea in women after laparoscopic gynaecological surgery. *Acta Anaesthesiol Scand* 2001;**45**:495–500.

34. Strayer RJ, Nelson LS. Adverse events associated with ketamine for procedural sedation in adults. *Am J Emerg Med* 2008;**26**:985–1028.

35. Friedberg BL. Propofol-ketamine technique. *Aesthetic Plast Surg* 1993;**17**:297–300.

36. Friedberg BL. Propofol ketamine anesthesia for cosmetic surgery in the office suite. *Int Anesthesiol Clin* 2003;**41**:39–50.

37. Messenger DW, Murray HE, Dungey PE, et al. Subdissociative-dose ketamine versus fentanyl for analgesia during propofol procedural sedation: a randomized clinical trial. *Acad Emerg Med* 2008;**15**:877–86.

38. Aouad MT, Moussa AR, Dagher CM, et al. Addition of ketamine to propofol for initiation of procedural anesthesia in children reduces propofol consumption and preserves hemodynamic stability. *Acta Anaesthesiol Scand* 2008;**52**:561–5.

39. Aouad MT, Moussa AR, Dagher CM, et al. Addition of ketamine to propofol for initiation of procedural anesthesia in children reduces propofol consumption and preserves hemodynamic stability. *Acta Anaesthesiol Scand* 2008;**52**:561–5.

40. Goel S, Bhardwaj N, Jain K. Efficacy of ketamine and midazolam as co-induction agents with propofol for laryngeal mask

insertion in children. *Paediatr Anaesth* 2008;**18**:628–34.

41. Slavik VC, Zed PJ. Combination ketamine and propofol for procedural sedation and analgesia. *Pharmacotherapy* 2007;**27**:1588–98.

42. De Kock MF, Lavand'homme PM. The clinical role of NMDA receptor antagonists for the treatment of postoperative pain. *Best Pract Res Clin Anaesthesiol* 2007;**21**:85–98.

43. Stubhaug A, Breivik H, Eide PK, et al. Mapping of punctuate hyperalgesia around a surgical incision demonstrates that ketamine is a powerful suppressor of central sensitization to pain following surgery. *Acta Anaesthesiol Scand* 1997;**41**:1124–32.

44. Bell RF, Dahl JB, Moore RA, Kalso E. Peri-operative ketamine for acute post-operative pain: a quantitative and qualitative systematic review (Cochrane review). *Acta Anaesthesiol Scand* 2005;**49**:1405–28.

45. Elia N, Tramèr MR. Ketamine and postoperative pain – a quantitative systematic review of randomised trials. *Pain* 2005;**113**:61–70.

46. Kwok RF, Lim J, Chan MT, et al. Preoperative ketamine improves postoperative analgesia after gynecologic laparoscopic surgery. *Anesth Analg* 2004;**98**:1044–9, table.

47. Roytblat L, Korotkoruchko A, Katz J, et al. Postoperative pain: the effect of low-dose ketamine in addition to general anesthesia. *Anesth Analg* 1993;**77**:1161–5.

48. Mathisen LC, Aasbo V, Raeder J. Lack of pre-emptive analgesic effect of (*R*)-ketamine in laparoscopic cholecystectomy. *Acta Anaesthesiol Scand* 1999;**43**:220–4.

49. Collard V, Mistraletti G, Taqi A, et al. Intraoperative esmolol infusion in the absence of opioids spares postoperative fentanyl in patients undergoing ambulatory laparoscopic cholecystectomy. *Anesth Analg* 2007;**105**:1255–62, table.

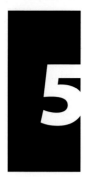

Anesthetic techniques for ambulatory surgery

General anesthesia

General anesthesia with modern agents has a record of very good safety, rapid onset, rapid offset, rapid emergence, and ease of administration [1]. A general anesthetic can be achieved with inhalational or intravenous techniques, or a combination of the two [2].

Inhalational anesthesia

Even though the pungency of sevoflurane is low and its action rapid, inhalational induction is not very popular in adults and its use has also declined in children due to the ease of intravenous (iv) line establishment using "eutectic mixture of local anesthetics (EMLA®)" cream. Also there is the possibility of probably harmless seizure-like EEG activity with high-dose sevoflurane in children [3] and a significant incidence of bothersome emergence agitation after sevoflurane termination in children [4]. However, there are centers that routinely use sevoflurane for induction of ambulatory patients [5], and the inhalational technique should always be a part of our armamentarium. It is excellent for adults with needle phobia and for children with difficult veins or poor cooperation. Sevoflurane is the best of the potent agents for inhalational induction. There is less airway irritation and a more rapid sequence when compared with desflurane or isoflurane. Halothane may work for induction, but is rather slow in onset and offset, and has been almost abandoned in western countries due to a rare but potentially lethal occurrence of halothane hepatitis in adults [6].

Inhalational anesthesia is mostly used for maintenance of anesthesia after an iv induction. Inhalational agents are easy to administer and easy to monitor, as online breath-by-breath monitoring of the end-tidal concentration, which is in fairly good equilibration with the effect site in the brain, is possible. However, there will be some shunting, even in the healthy young lung when lying down, more so in the elderly and the obese, and even more with prolonged procedures. This shunting will cause the end-tidal values to be 5–30% higher than mixed-arterial values during induction, and 5–20% lower than arterial values during emergence. With a facial mask or a loose laryngeal mask airway (LMA) there may be admittance of room air into the system, causing the end-tidal measurement to be lower than arterial levels during both induction and emergence.

The risk of overdose and accumulation with inhalational agents is relatively low as there is no accumulation beyond the concentration set by the vaporizer, and end-tidal monitoring also ensures control of the actual level in the patient. When using re-breathing and low-flow systems the drug costs are generally lower than with total intravenous (TIVA) techniques. The investment costs of the equipment (i.e., vaporizer, scavenger, room ventilation, etc.) are higher than with TIVA techniques and the equipment is bulkier to transport into rooms or areas not dedicated for inhalational anesthesia, such as a diagnostic room or an office-based unit. Inhalational agents provide better patient-maintained respiration and more rapid, immediate, emergence when compared to propofol [7]. This difference in emergence is only evident during the first 5–15 min after procedures of short or intermediate duration [8], and is presently challenged by techniques using remifentanil combined with propofol. Especially when the drugs are tapered down by the end of surgery, any modern technique may render the patient awake and communicating with the staff within 2–5 min. For procedures lasting more than 2–3 hours there seems to be a benefit with desflurane [9] in terms of faster emergence and also better respiration at equipotent doses when compared with sevoflurane. Desflurane seems to result in less emergence agitation than sevoflurane, and, for this reason, some pediatric anesthesiologists choose to switch to desflurane for maintenance after a sevoflurane inhalational induction [10]. There is an increased incidence of shivering [11] and postoperative nausea and vomiting (PONV) [12] after potent inhalational agents, the latter especially with isoflurane or desflurane [13], when compared with propofol [14]. This has been disputed in some recent studies showing less shivering after desflurane compared with propofol [15,16].

Nitrous oxide [2]

Although its use is controversial due to possible toxic effects, pollution, and nausea, nitrous oxide continues to be popular as an adjunct to either total intravenous anesthesia (TIVA; it may be semantically disputed whether TIVA with nitrous oxide can still be called TIVA!) or potent inhalational anesthetics. The popularity is due to its rapid offset even after prolonged administration, and the almost complete absence of both respiratory and circulatory depression in the healthy. Nitrous oxide has a combined analgesic + hypnotic action, reducing the need for other anesthetics [17]. The role of nitrous oxide as a cause of PONV has been controversial and debated. In a meta-analysis the conclusion was that nitrous oxide may contribute to PONV when the baseline risk is high, but otherwise not [18]. One problem with nitrous oxide relates to the evolving regulations of the levels allowed in the operating theater air to minimize risk to the personnel working there. As with other inhalational anesthetics, cumbersome and expensive equipment is needed for safe administration and scavenging, adding to investment costs. These should be balanced against the low running cost of the agent.

Intravenous anesthesia

Any routine iv induction agent may be used, such as a barbiturate, etomidate, propofol, and, in the rare cases of severe hypovolemia, ketamine with a benzodiazepine. Propofol is considered by most to be the cornerstone of modern ambulatory general anesthesia due to its associated rapid and clearheaded recovery, most often with a pleasant almost euphoric mood, combined with some initial protection against nausea and vomiting. In order to dose more precisely in a simplified way, the commercial target control infusion (TCI) system Diprifusor® has become increasingly popular, especially after the release of different models for dosing and the possibility of using generic preparations and syringes (see Target control infusion, Chapter 4). Instead of the usual way of dosing in milligrams per kilogram, the TCI algorithm controls the pump rate to deliver a chosen plasma or CNS concentration to the patient and adjusts infusion to maintain a stable concentration despite ongoing distribution out of the blood and elimination. Nevertheless, the benefit of this system has been disputed. The algorithm is not very accurate [19], and it has been shown that a good clinician may achieve similar accuracy and better total economy using manual infusion schemes [20].

Opioids

Opioids are used in general anesthesia together with propofol in most cases when nociceptive stimulation from tissue trauma is anticipated. Many will also prefer to use some opioid together with inhalational agents in order to reduce the consumption of gas and to provide analgesia on emergence. The difference between the modern potent peroperative opioids seems to be in their pharmacokinetic characteristics, as their side-effect profiles at equi-analgesic effect levels seem to be similar. In terms of onset, sufentanil and fentanyl are slower than alfentanil and remifentanil. In terms of duration of effect the context-sensitive elimination half-time should be considered, as should the dosing level. Care should be taken in particular not to use high doses of fentanyl, as this may slow down recovery and increase the incidence of PONV. However, small doses (i.e., 0.5–1.0 µg/kg) of fentanyl are quite short lasting (20–30 min) and excellent for avoiding or controlling immediate postoperative pain.

Remifentanil is very well suited for ambulatory care owing to its rapid onset, similar to that of alfentanil, and an unrivalled rapid clearance within minutes, even after large doses or prolonged administration. Questions have been raised as to whether these potent opioids, especially remifentanil, may induce acute tolerance and even hyperalgesia with increased postoperative need for analgesics after a few hours of infusion or repeated administration [21–23]. With moderate doses (i.e., remifentanil at 0.1–0.2 µg/kg per minute) for up to 1–2 hours of administration, the hyperalgesia does not seem to be abundant or long lasting (Lenz et al., submitted 2010). This contrasts with the required dose in the range of 0.3–0.5 µg/kg per minute, for instance as needed for cruciate ligament repair, where a need for high-dose opioids postoperatively may be even higher due to hyperalgesia [24]. In an experimental model in which only 0.1 µg/kg per minute of remifentanil for 30 min was given to volunteers, there was a minor but significant hyperalgesia for 1–2 h afterwards (Lenz et al., submitted 2010).

Neuromuscular block, intubation

The use of neuromuscular blocking agents has definitely declined in modern ambulatory surgery. Almost all patients sent for ambulatory surgery have an empty stomach and the surgery case mix consists mainly of procedures that do not require profound muscle relaxation. Nevertheless, there are cases where a 100% assurance of immobility is needed (e.g., some eye surgery, ear surgery, micro-surgery). Decreased use of endotracheal intubation is also the result of the increased popularity of the LMA [25]. It has been shown that the LMA is less traumatic during introduction and reduces postoperative sore throat compared with endotracheal intubation [25]. A tight, well-fitting LMA probably protects the larynx and airways against aspiration of small volumes of fluid from the stomach or oropharynx, but with large volumes of aspirate a cuffed endotracheal tube is more reliable. By using an LMA model with inbuilt gastric tube facilities (e.g., the ProSeal™), the stomach may be safely drained of both fluids and accidental gas influx from the peritoneal cavity, as may very rarely occur for instance during laparoscopic procedures.

There are cases when many anesthetists prefer to have an endotracheal tube in place for safety reasons (e.g., tonsillectomy, extensive laparoscopy) or for more reliable ventilation, as in obese patients. With modern potent short-acting drugs (i.e., propofol and alfentanil or remifentanil) and perhaps the additional use of local anesthetic spray, endotracheal intubation may be accomplished without neuromuscular blockade.

A bolus dose of 3–4 μg/kg remifentanil given slowly over 2–3 min during or after induction of sleep with propofol will ensure sufficiently profound analgesia and relaxation of the vocal cords to allow for endotracheal intubation. Care should be taken not to give the full dose of remifentanil before any hypnotic agent is given (i.e., propofol or midazolam), as a stiff chest may occur in the otherwise drug-naive patient with doses beyond 1 μg/kg of remifentanil as a rapid bolus. A hypnotic dose of propofol seems to protect almost completely against a stiff chest, then even bolus doses of 3–4 μg/kg remifentanil seem to work smoothly. Still many anesthetists prefer to use a nondepolarizing neuromuscular blocker for intubation, and also surgeons may prefer to have relaxation present during their dissection (see also Chapter 4). A single dose of cisatracurium (0.08 mg/kg) or rocuronium (0.6 mg/kg) will usually do, both for intubation and surgery. If the train of four (TOF) shows at least 90% recovery by the end of the procedure, there is no need for neostigmine reversal. As neostigmine is associated with a dose-related increased risk of PONV, non-reversal may be of benefit. If the TOF is less than 90%, a dose of up to 2.5 mg neostigmine with glycopyrrolate should be used. If the block is profound (fewer than two twitches on TOF) it may be an indication to use sugammadex 2 mg/kg for rapid and complete reversal. Sugammadex only works for reversal of rocuronium or vecuronium and is very expensive. As a smaller dose (0.25–0.5 mg/kg) may be sufficient for reversal of blocks with one to two twitches, and may be given together with neostigmine, economy may be improved by using one ampoule for more than one patient. Suxamethonium is the optimal relaxant in terms of rapid onset and short duration, but the side-effects of muscle pain and occasional anaphylaxis may be a problem. Mivacurium is a nondepolarizing alternative with spontaneous degradation within 20–30 min, but, like suxamethonium, rare genetic degradation failure may be seen.

Regional and local anesthesia

Regional anesthesia may be defined as anesthetizing a smaller or larger region by local anesthetics applied to major nerves, trunks, or nerve bundles innervating the surgical area. Regional anesthesia may be further divided into nerve blocks and central neuraxial blocks, i.e., spinal or epidural anesthesia. This is as opposed to *local anesthesia*, where the local anesthetics are applied (i.e., infiltrated, splashed, smeared) directly into the surgical area, acting on small, peripheral nerve fibers and receptors. There are some transition areas between local anesthesia and regional anesthesia, such as finger blocks, para-cervical block, or eye blocks, where both major nerve block and the localized small fiber action may be involved. Regional and local anesthesia methods also use the same drugs and share many of the same benefits and potential problems, thus they are often discussed together as loco-regional techniques. They may be used as (1) the only anesthetic provided, (2) together with sedation, or (3) as a supplement to general anesthesia. In US literature the term "monitored anesthesia care" or MAC, is used for surgical procedures carried out under local anesthesia combined with anesthesiologic sedation.

Loco-regional techniques are well suited for ambulatory surgery owing to their potential for less postoperative nausea and pain combined with less sedation and possibly less cognitive dysfunction [26]. The different techniques should be used with the focus being on providing minimal preoperative delays and fast discharge-readiness, while maintaining the benefits they afford.

Why should we use loco-regional techniques for ambulatory anesthesia?

Safety

The ambulatory setting has a high focus on safety, rapid emergence, and good control of postoperative pain. In this context, loco-regional techniques have good potential: minimal generalized drug effects, option of being awake during the procedure, and superior pain control immediately after the procedure [27]. However, the ideal of zero mortality and no permanent disability after ambulatory care [28] has been challenged by reports of rare, but serious, complications of permanent nerve damage [29], spinal hematomas, and spinal or general toxicity [30]. In a report from France, 56 major complications were reported after loco-regional anesthesia in a mixed population of 158 000 inpatients and outpatients [31]. These included 9 cardiac arrest cases during spinal anesthesia and 12 cases of probably permanent nerve damage after peripheral blocks. Most of these reports were from seriously ill or unstable inpatients. A low quality in the practice of local anesthesia and sedation in ambulatory care was associated with a higher mortality following liposuction in Florida [32].

Quality

Better postoperative pain control remains a major issue for improvement after surgery [33], and loco-regional techniques have consistently proved beneficial in this context [33,34]. As loco-regional analgesia for surgery is established before initiation of the surgical trauma, there is also the potential to exploit the disputed benefits of pre-emptive analgesia with fewer pain-generating reflexes into the central nervous system (see Chapter 6).

No inhalational drugs and fewer opioid analgesics are needed when loco-regional techniques are used, therefore a lower incidence of PONV is usually seen when these techniques are compared with general anesthesia [35].

The perioperative setting and choice of technique may have an impact on the incidence of impaired cognitive function postoperatively, which is reported with a higher frequency in elderly patients and after major surgery [36]. When regional anesthesia was compared with general anesthesia in a prospective, randomized way, there was less impairment ($P<0.05$) at 1 week after regional techniques, whereas the figures at 3 months were similar [37].

With loco-regional techniques there is the option for the patient to be fully awake during the procedure. It may be interesting and educational for the patient in some cases to watch the endoscopy screen or talk with the surgeon about their findings, measures, and plans for postoperative behavior. For the surgeon it may sometimes be helpful to discuss the details of symptoms with the patient while the anatomy is revealed on the screen. Having the patient awake will, of course, put some demand on all members of the operating room team to keep the conversation appropriate and to focus on creating a reassuring atmosphere for the patient. An alternative or adjunct may be to have an awake patient wearing headphones listening to music. With a non-stressful situation the patient may be well off with any of their favorite music, but in situations filled with much stress or anxiety it may be better to play neutral, unfamiliar music in order to avoid recall of the events if the particular music piece is played later in life.

Most patients prefer some kind of sedation. In terms of giving the patient peroperative instructions it should be kept in mind that even low doses of benzodiazepines or propofol will result in amnesia, whereas an opioid-based technique may not. Sedation during loco-regional techniques may be indicated because of pain, patient anxiety, or according to patient preference, and choice of agent should be guided by the specific needs of the individual patient (see later, Sedation). However, use of sedation may have side-effects. In a study of loco-regional patients with either propofol or remifentanil sedation, Servin et al. showed more respiratory depression and peroperative nausea with remifentanil, and more peroperative pain and delayed emergence with propofol [38].

For minor anxiolysis a small dose of diazepam (2.5–5 mg) may be appropriate, although anxiolysis combined with a hypnotic effect may be more reliably achieved by midazolam 1–2 mg, which may be repeated once or twice. More extensive dosing of benzodiazepines should be avoided, as this may delay recovery. Otherwise propofol sedation may be very easily titrated: a small dose for anxiolysis (which will also cause amnesia), somewhat more for sleep, and if needed a smooth and rapid conversion to general anesthesia by increasing the dose together with an opioid and eventually respiratory support and laryngeal mask. If pain is an indication for sedation, the primary choice of remifentanil may be more appropriate, but care should be taken to examine for (and treat!) any nausea and respiratory depression.

Dexmedetomidine is a very interesting new alternative α2 agonist sedative drug. It seems to have a minor respiratory depressive effect and combines analgesic and sedative hypnotic effects to induce a state that resembles normal sleep; there is a very rapid and clearheaded transition between sleep and awake states. It is becoming popular in the pediatric setting [39], although it seems that recovery in adults may be prolonged when compared with conventional methods [40].

Efficacy, economy

Better total economy is one of the driving forces behind the development of ambulatory surgery, and regional anesthetic drugs are usually cheaper than their general anesthetic counterparts.

The concept of fast-tracking, i.e., direct transfer of the patient from the operating room to phase-II step-down recovery, bypassing the postanesthesia care unit (PACU), has evolved successfully with loco-regional techniques [41]. In a US survey of five centers, 90% of all cases receiving MAC (i.e. local anesthesia with iv sedation) were fast-tracked compared with 32% of cases with general anesthesia [42]. Such comparisons are not always totally fair, as the case mix often varies, with less extensive procedures being done under local anesthesia. Furthermore, increased delays until establishment of regional block and delayed recovery due to urinary retention or paralyzed legs after spinal anesthesia remain major challenges for these techniques in the ambulatory setting [27]. In a recent British survey of practice in 270 departments for either day-case cystoscopy or knee arthroscopy, all the respondents used general anesthesia as their major method, although supplements of local anesthesia were used by 26% for cystoscopy and 77% for knee arthroscopy [43].

The increased time for block establishment and prolonged bed rest or urinary retention after spinal blocks should be added into the drug cost calculation, as should an uneventful recovery with less nausea and pain. The net economic balance will vary according to the local circumstances. In a study of desflurane versus spinal anesthesia for hysteroscopy, the latter was cheaper [44], whereas Danelli et al. found no difference in total economy when spinal anesthesia was compared with general anesthesia for hysteroscopies [45]. In studies of MAC with local anesthesia and sedation, this technique is usually favorable in terms of total economy [46].

New drugs, equipment, and methods

Drugs

Ropivacaine and *levobupivacaine* have been launched as less toxic alternatives to *bupivacaine*. Whereas levobupivacaine is very similar and equipotent to racemic bupivacaine, ropivacaine seems to be slightly less potent in most applications. Further, ropivacaine seems to have a better separation between motor and sensory block, and has been approved for spinal use and continuous post-operative nerve block infusion. However, there is still ongoing debate as to whether the increased cost of these new drugs used routinely is justified by their potential clinical safety benefits [47].

Articaine and preservative-free *2-chloroprocaine* have been launched as short-acting alternatives to lidocaine for spinal anesthesia, without the risk of benign transient neurologic symptoms (TNS), which are often seen after lidocaine.

Experimentally, there are potential local anesthetic drugs capable of blocking c-fibers selectively, and also capsaicin-like drugs may have a potential in this direction [48].

For many years there has also been pre-license work on slow-release local anesthetic drugs or drug formulations with effects lasting for 1–2 days after single-dose infiltration, but so far none of these formulas has been approved for clinical use.

Equipment

A major breakthrough in making regional nerve blocks more interesting, easier, and safer has been the development of ultrasound imaging of nerves and their surrounding anatomic structures. With noninvasive ultrasound the needle can be placed very close to the nerve with less risk of very rare nerve damage, as with paresthesia techniques, and also without causing the patient the discomfort of jerking during electrical nerve stimulation [49]. Furthermore, the precise positioning of the needle tip allows for a lower dose to be used and thus a reduced risk of systemic toxicity; there is also less tissue pressure from a high-volume injection, which may occasionally be suspected to result in ischemia and nerve compression. The success rate will also increase with more precise needle positioning. As the spread of local anesthetic drug may be seen on the screen, the anesthetist will be able to spot cases where minor connective tissue septa stop the normal distribution of local anesthetic drug.

Ultrasound devices are very expensive to buy and training is needed in order to use them successfully. Thus, for small units and units where regional blocks are not performed regularly, or for doctors who do not do blocks frequently, there will still be a place for conventional nerve stimulation and even paresthesia techniques.

An interesting area of refined use of equipment is prolonged infusion or repeated bolus dosing of local anesthetic into wounds or joints. This may be just a single dose at the end of surgery but may be extended to the patient's self-care at home for some days after ambulatory surgery, as reported by Rawal [50] and others [51]. Ropivacaine (2 mg/ml) seems to be the drug of choice, due to its low toxicity, as either infusions with disposable elastomeric pumps or bolus injections at 4- to 6-h intervals. A special situation is the patient with a wound drain, where infusions may pass directly into the drainage without having any effect. In those cases a bolus technique may be appropriate: close the drains, give a bolus, keep drains closed for 30 min and then re-open the drains [52].

New techniques

Although not actually new, there is great and renewed interest in the refinement of high-volume (i.e., 100–300 ml) dosing with low concentrations of local anesthetic, infiltrated extensively by the surgeon at the end of surgery, i.e., local infiltration anesthesia (LIA). Usually mixtures of 1–2 mg/ml of levobupivacaine or ropivacaine are used, sometimes combined with opioid, clonidine, ketamine, and/or NSAIDS. Most reports to date are in the field of major orthopedic surgery [53].

What are the prerequisites for successful loco-regional use in ambulatory care?

Accepted by the surgeon

If the surgeon is unwilling or not cooperative during loco-regional anesthesia, the chance of problems and failure will increase significantly. Sometimes it may simply be a matter of providing the surgeon with better information about the benefits of loco-regional anesthesia or discussing the option of providing adequate sedation in order to let the surgeon work undisturbed. In other cases the surgeon may have valid concerns about muscle relaxation and surgical access, or the surgeon and patient may have made alternative plans in their prior consultations.

Accepted by the patient

Patients who do not consent to loco-regional anesthesia, even after full discussion of the technique, should not be forced into it, unless strong contraindications to general anesthesia are present (see later). Nevertheless, it is wise to spend time with reluctant patients, first stating that their opinions will be heard, then presenting the pros and cons of their treatment options, and ending by stating what method is normally used in cases such as theirs. For reluctant patients it is often useful to emphasize that a strong analgesic (i.e., small bolus of alfentanil or remifentanil) will be given before any painful needles and that once the block has been tested and found to be effective, there is no problem in ensuring 100% sleep (i.e., propofol) during the procedure on top of the block. Once a decision has been taken, it is important for all personnel to back it and to be supportive and friendly, not trying to persuade a review of the decision or signaling that they disapprove in any way.

For both surgeons and patients it is reassuring and positive to know whether the loco-regional technique is used routinely by the team for the specific procedure and type of patient in question; it is also good to remember that "routine" never means "always," and that exceptions will be made from time to time.

Avoid preoperative delay

With some blocks, such as paracervical blocks and spinal anesthesia, administration and onset take no longer than general anesthesia induction. However with other blocks, such as epidural anesthesia and brachial plexus blocks, the administration of the block may take time, testing takes time, and failure may occur, especially in inexperienced hands or with obese patients. The use of a separate induction room to prepare the blocks may be an advantage, especially in units with anesthetists in training or where operating room (OR) availability creates a bottle-neck in the treatment chain. If an induction room is not an option, the block has to be done in the OR. An effective measure then is to automatically assume that the block will be effective. The implication of this is that the patient can be immediately placed in position, washed, and draped as soon as the block is done. Usually these procedures are carried out while the plexus block takes effect, and a rapid test of block efficacy may be done using the surgeon's forceps immediately before the start of surgery. In rare cases (a benchmark goal should be less than 1 case out of 10–20) of insufficient block, a very low threshold should be set for immediately starting propofol and opioid, perhaps with an LMA to induce general anesthesia within 2–3 min, before starting the operation.

Some tricks may also be used to make the local anesthetic work faster: body-temperature local anesthetic works faster than cold and lidocaine's action may be hastened by adding 0.5 mmol/ml Na-bicarbonate. It is disputed whether adrenaline adjunct speeds up onset, and opioid adjunct may actually slow it down by lowering the pH.

Ensure a low block failure rate

This comes with training and experience, but may be challenged by time constraint and a stressful working environment. Induction rooms may lower the failure rate, as does the use of good equipment such as nerve stimulators and, in particular, appropriate ultrasound imaging and experience in its use. It is recommended that every anesthetist has a limited repertoire of basic blocks that they are able to implement frequently (see later on, "my choices") instead of a large variety of blocks, each seldom used.

Avoid prolonged block (?)

A prolonged neuraxial block may delay recovery and discharge due to prolonged leg paralysis and occasionally complications such as urinary retention, but it will also ensure prolonged analgesia. For ambulatory surgery these neuraxial blocks should be done with short-lasting drugs, unless a prolonged surgical procedure is anticipated. A better strategy though for potentially prolonged procedures is to use short-acting drugs, but insert a catheter in case repeated dosing becomes necessary.

For nerve blocks with a limited area of paralysis it may be totally advantageous to have a prolonged block, because pain protection is better and longer lasting. If the patient has been given appropriate information it is usually acceptable to discharge a patient with a paralyzed arm in a sling or a paralyzed foot within a bandage or plaster.

Which procedures are appropriate for local anesthesia?

The very simple but also current and correct answer to this question is that ALL surgical procedures should receive optimal local anesthesia infiltration, independently of whether the local anesthesia technique is the only anesthetic, the major anesthetic (i.e., together with some sedation), an important peroperative adjuvant, or an important component of post-operative analgesic strategy. The surgeon may use local anesthesia before the start of surgery or during surgery as they cut into new structures. Often a rapid-acting drug, such as lidocaine, is used for this purpose. In these cases it may be advisable to supplement with long-acting local anesthetics at the end of the procedure in order to optimize postoperative analgesia. Pavlin et al. reported a 32% reduction in postoperative opioid consumption when local wound anesthesia was used in a mixed case list of ambulatory surgery [33].

In some cases it may be argued that preoperative infiltration may alter the anatomy and worsen surgical access. Also, local anesthetic may be removed along with dissected tissue or diffuse into blood and fluids in the surgical field, but these possibilities should not discourage the surgeon from infiltrating local anesthetic by the end of the procedure.

Local anesthesia is often unsuitable for major surgery, either because it has an insufficient ability to block all relevant pain structures, or because too high a dose is needed and toxicity

Table 5.1. Local anesthesia for infiltration: Concentration, onset, duration, maximum dose[a] (single)

Drug	Concentration (mg/ml)	Onset	Duration	Maximal dose (mg/kg)[b]
Lidocaine	5–20	Fast	Medium	10
Mepivacaine	5–20	Fast	Medium+	10
Bupivacaine	2.5–5	Medium	Long	2.5
Levobupivacaine	2.5–5	Medium	Long	4
Ropivacaine	2–7.5	Medium	Long	3.5

[a] Will always depend on the potential for rapid diffusion of a large amount into the circulation, weighed against the potential for side-effects with each drug.
[b] The maximum dose may be increased when adrenaline adjunct is used and also when there is infiltration into a large area with a minor risk of the full dose coming into circulation (major vessels) at the same time.

results from extensive infiltration. This view has been challenged by the concept of LIA (see above), in which a low concentration of lidocaine or ropivacaine (down to 2 or 1 mg/ml, respectively) may allow 100–150 ml to infiltrate extensively.

However, for intermediate and minor surgical procedures being done under ambulatory care, stronger concentrations in appropriate and smaller volumes can be used. Local anesthesia is simple and cheap, and provides excellent postoperative pain relief [27]. A study of local anesthesia for inguinal hernia repair showed the technique to be favorable compared with general or spinal anesthesia [54] and this is also supported in an editorial and by a large patient study from Denmark [55]. The utilization of local anesthesia has increasing potential as many surgical procedures are becoming less invasive as the result of new technology and skills. Examples of this development are reports of local anesthesia use during both vaginal taping for stress incontinence [56] and sentinel node biopsies for breast cancer [57].

Care should be taken to respect the maximal safe doses of local anesthetic drugs and there is a preference to replace bupivacaine with the less toxic ropivacaine or levobupivacaine whenever more than 1–2 mg/kg is used (see Table 5.1).

Which procedures are appropriate for regional anesthesia?

In general all procedures that may be performed with regional anesthesia for inpatients may be done the same way in the ambulatory setting. These include all procedures on the extremities, including shoulder arthroscopic surgery. Regional anesthesia may be used in all surgical procedures beneath the umbilicus, including low laparotomies and most gynecologic procedures. Superficial procedures on the trunk (plastic surgery, breast surgery) may also be performed with regional anesthesia or local infiltration. Some regions are not suited for regional anesthesia, such as the upper abdomen or thorax. Although there is no "true" regional block for procedures on the head, face, and neck, surgery in this region may often be performed with nerve blocks and infiltration. For procedures involving more than one region simultaneously (e.g., skin transplantation), loco-regional techniques may be used at one or both sites. Care must be taken to obey the upper limits for dosing to avoid toxicity.

What are the contraindications to loco-regional anesthesia?

- Patients who do not consent (see above).

- For patients with nerve injury or neurologic deficit in the area of planned block, it is a good general rule to avoid loco-regional techniques. Although loco-regional anesthesia has not been shown to worsen any neurologic deficit, it may be wise to avoid the potential for speculation and discussion with the patient afterwards about these issues. This means that if there is a good indication for loco-regional anesthesia, if general anesthesia presents problems, or if the patient is otherwise motivated to have such an approach, it may well be done. In any case, it is wise to assess neurologic function before applying the anesthesia, and also to document the discussion with the patient and the decision made before going ahead.

- Uncooperative patients may be poor subjects for loco-regional anesthesia. Again, the contraindication is relative and must be weighed against the alternatives. A feasible approach in special cases may be to induce hypnosis with a modest dose of propofol, and then do the block, preferably with a nerve stimulator or ultrasound, and not in a region (e.g., high epidural) where communication with the patient is important. Uncooperative children and elderly patients in particular may actually profit from loco-regional techniques due to the excellent postoperative analgesia they afford.

- Infection at the site of the block is an absolute contraindication. Also a tattoo may be a relative contraindication if the needle has to go directly through a pigmented skin area. Such pigments may be drawn in with the needle tip and become neurotoxic. This concern is most valid with spinal anesthesia and the problem can usually be managed by moving the needle a few millimeters to a skin spot without pigmentation.

- Anticoagulated patients should be evaluated more strictly for neuraxial blocks in the outpatient setting than as inpatients. A postoperative hematoma developing after discharge is more dangerous in terms of diagnosis and delays from pressure ischemia or nerve tissue injury than it is in a carefully observed inpatient.

Neuraxial blocks for ambulatory anesthesia

Epidural anesthesia

There are few recent reports in the literature on epidural anesthesia for ambulatory care. Epidural anesthesia is usually regarded as more time consuming compared with other techniques. Our data on epidural anesthesia with mepivacaine showed discharge readiness after 2 h, whereas that after a lidocaine spinal was about 30 min less [58]. A study by Mulroy and co-workers actually showed a faster discharge, namely about 2 h after surgery, with epidural block with either lidocaine or 2-chloroprocaine when compared with spinal lidocaine or low-dose bupivacaine [59]. In another study of 256 hemorrhoidectomy patients, either 20 ml lidocaine 1% or bupivacaine 0.5% epidurally was used, but the observation time in hospital was a minimum of 5 h and 2% of the patients were admitted due to urinary retention [60]. In a study of lower body surgery, epidural administration of 16 ml lidocaine 1.6% was used, but all the patients were observed for 6 h in the hospital [61]. Although epidural needles are thick and some outpatients used NSAIDs or had a history of bruising, epidural steroid injections caused no hematoma in a mixed population of 1035 patients [62]. However, a recent case report told of a 35-year-old woman with no risk factors, apart from peroperative ketorolac administration, who developed an epidural hematoma after discharge from an ambulatory arthroscopy under epidural anesthesia [63].

My choice for the very rare epidural anesthesia for adult surgery in the ambulatory setting will be an 18 G needle, loss of resistance with saline, and lumbar catheter placement, starting with 15–20 ml of either plain lidocaine or mepivacaine (20 mg/ml) in an adult. In children a caudal epidural may, in contrast to adults, more often be relevant for postoperative pain relief; a 21 G needle through the hiatus membrane, careful aspiration to rule out blood, and then application of ropivacaine (2 mg/kg; 0.5–1.5 ml/kg).

Paravertebral anesthesia

Paravertebral anesthesia is a unilateral alternative to epidural anesthesia with prolonged postoperative pain relief. It has been used successfully for ambulatory breast surgery [64] and inguinal hernia repair [65]. In a study using paravertebral ropivacaine for hernia repair, the average time for block administration was 12 min and analgesia was provided for 15 h, which was significantly better than with local infiltration block with ropivacaine [66]. However, in a series of 30 patients, there were two cases of block failure and two cases of prolonged recovery due to epidural effects [65].

Unilateral paravertebral anesthesia may be an excellent choice alone or as an adjunct to sedation for breast cancer surgery. In one study the data actually indicated a lower incidence of cancer relapse after this block, although some confounders could be present from the nonrandomized retrospective design [67]. In any case, there seems to be better initial pain relief after this block and minor side-effects, at least after moderate or more extensive procedures [68].

My choice would be an 18 G epidural needle, 2.5 cm from the midline, aiming to hit the transverse spike of the fourth or fifth thoracic vertebra, then adjusting the needle to pass above the spike, and moving it further in (1–2 cm) until loss of resistance. I give either 25–30 ml of 5 mg/kg ropivacaine in this one shot covering four to five dermatomes, or I inject 15 ml into this location and make a new deposit of 15 ml three to four levels down.

Spinal anesthesia

Spinal anesthesia is popular for ambulatory patients in some units, whereas in others neuraxial blocks are not used at all. Some major controversies here are reviewed by Salinas and Liu [69].

As ambulatory patients are mobilized and prone to feel symptoms of a spinal headache, a thin (i.e., 27 G) needle of pencil point design should be used and the incidence of mild headache is expected to be less than 1–2% and even lower in the elderly or obese patients. Theoretically 29 G needles should be even better in this respect, but in clinical use they are more difficult to direct and spinal flow is so low that there is a risk of multiple dura puncture and also failure.

The occurrence of transient neurologic symptoms (TNS) has been associated particularly with ambulatory surgery (rapid mobilization), the lithotomy position, or manipulation of the hip joint during knee arthroscopy, and almost exclusively with lidocaine [69]. TNS is a benign and self-limiting condition, but in a study by Tong et al. the patients with TNS had more pain during the first 72 h after surgery and reduced activities of daily living for 24 h compared with the patients without TNS [70]. Variation of the lidocaine concentration or hyperbaricity seems to have little influence on the incidence [70], but there seems to be a lower incidence when the lidocaine dose is reduced [69]. In a study of 36 patients with 25 mg lidocaine spinally, no TNS was observed [59]. However, in order for lidocaine doses of less than 40 mg to be effective, an opioid adjunct is usually needed [69]. In the study of

Buckenmaier et al. 20 µg fentanyl was added to 25 mg lidocaine for anorectal procedures [71], whereas Lennox et al. added sufentanil 10 µg to only 10 mg lidocaine for gynecologic laparoscopy [72]. In the latter study it seems as though anesthesia was on the lower threshold for acceptance, as 30% of the patients reported peroperative discomfort. However, motor recovery and discharge readiness were even faster than in a comparator group receiving desflurane anesthesia [72]. A mixture of lidocaine (20 mg) with fentanyl (20 µg) was sufficient for knee arthroscopy in the study of Ben-David et al. [29]. Another approach to avoid TNS is to use ropivacaine or bupivacaine. In studies of identical doses of these two drugs, either 12.5 mg [73] or 15 mg [74], there was no TNS. A conclusion in favor of ropivacaine was made, as motor block was less prominent and recovery faster compared with bupivacaine. This may be due to nonequipotency in dosing, as bupivacaine should probably be dosed lower than ropivacaine for equal effect [75]. Future studies are needed to clarify whether a clinical issue of less motor block and shorter recovery with ropivacaine at the minimal effective dose remains.

Bupivacaine for ambulatory spinal anesthesia is usually combined with an opioid to reduce the dose needed and the duration of motor block. With a combination of bupivacaine 15 mg + fentanyl 10 µg, 50–75% of patients had impairment of walking and standing for more than 90 min. This was in spite of a low incidence of motor block – fewer than 25% of the patients had measurable peroperative weakness in the leg musculature [76]. Urinary retention delayed average discharge by 30 min when spinal levobupivacaine (10 mg) or ropivacaine (15 mg) was compared with lidocaine (60 mg) [75]. In a study of hernia repair, Gupta et al. used fentanyl (25 µg) together with bupivacaine (either 6 mg or 7.5 mg) [77]. The 6 mg dose necessitated supplemental iv analgesia in some cases, and average discharge time was in range of 5–6 h in both groups. In this study, 17% of the patients needed catheterization, resulting in 5% being admitted overnight [77]. In a study of bupivacaine (10 mg) spinally for hysteroscopy, recovery and discharge were significantly longer than with remifentanil + propofol anesthesia [45].

It is debatable whether patients undergoing ambulatory surgery with spinal anesthesia can be discharged before voiding. Mulroy et al. claims that otherwise healthy patients less than 70 years old, with no history of voiding problems, and who are not undergoing surgery in the perianal or perineal region or having hernia repair may be discharged safely 2 h after bupivacaine (6 mg) spinally, even if they not have voided [59].

An approach for further bupivacaine dose reduction is to administer hyperbaric bupivacaine and then place the patient in the lateral decubitus position for 10–15 min to achieve unilateral spinal block. This was used successfully by Korhonen et al., who compared 4 mg bupivacaine with a mixture of 3 mg bupivacaine + 10 µg fentanyl for knee arthroscopy [78]. Of the two, the latter group had a higher rate of fast-tracking and their recovery unit stay was shorter, but discharge-readiness was similar in both groups, with a mean value of 3 h [78]. A major problem with opioid adjunct to spinal anesthesia is the high frequency of pruritus, at an incidence of 25–75% [69,78]. With a combination of iv droperidol (0.625 mg) and nalbuphine (4 mg), Ben-David et al. were able to reduce significantly the incidence of both pruritus and nausea, without provoking any more pain [29]. Another interesting adjunct is clonidine, which was optimally dosed at 15 µg with better block quality and no delay in recovery (i.e., about 2 h) when added to 8 mg ropivacaine [79]. Merivirta and co-workers added clonidine 15 µg to 5 mg unilateral bupivacaine, and found an increased need for initial vasopressors with clonidine, but a better block quality, and no delay in discharge-readiness [80].

A simpler and promising development in ambulatory spinal anesthesia is the launch of new, safe, short-acting local anesthetic agents. Articaine 50 mg was shown to provide discharge-readiness within 3 h, significantly faster than prilocaine [81], and 40–50 mg of 2-chloroprocaine seems even faster with ambulation and discharge-readiness within 2 h [82].

My choice depends somewhat on the case, but I always use a 27 G pencil point needle. For a unilateral leg procedure I will go with 5 mg bupivacaine and place the patient in the lateral position for 15 min. For a bilateral or perineal procedure I still go for lidocaine (20 mg/ml, 2–3 ml), with the needle hole pointing caudally, and inform the patient about the potential for mild, benign TNS. When 2-chloroprocaine (or articaine) is commercially available for spinal use, I will probably change to a 50 mg dose of this drug.

Use of peripheral blocks for ambulatory surgery

Peripheral blocks have the major advantage of not resulting in general hemodynamic changes to the same degree as neuraxial blocks. Furthermore, they may be achieved with long-acting drugs and even catheters, as full recovery from the block before patient discharge is usually not necessary and sometimes is not even beneficial.

Single lower extremity surgery

For single lower extremity surgery there are several choices of regional technique. In a study of 1200 knee-surgery patients, the combination of femoral and sciatic nerve block resulted in less pain and fewer hospital admissions than general anesthesia without block [83]. Although simple and efficacious for foot surgery, the ankle block technique is somewhat unreliable. Combined with a saphenous or femoral nerve block, posterior popliteal sciatic nerve block seems like a more reliable alternative. Several authors advocate the use of sciatic nerve block with different approaches. Provenzano et al. investigated the popliteal fossa nerve block supplemented with saphenous nerve block on 834 patients who underwent foot and/or ankle surgery [84]. In 80% of cases this technique was successful even when performed by anesthesiologists with little training. There were no incidents of postoperative neuralgia or neurapraxia. Using a different technique, Pandin et al. reports a remarkable no-failure rate for sciatic nerve block in the supine position [85]. Using landmarks somewhat higher up than the popliteal fossa and a nerve stimulator, these investigators were able to block the tibial and superficial peroneal nerves in 100% of cases, while the deep peroneal nerve and the postero-femoral cutaneous nerves were blocked in 97% and 83% of the patients, respectively [85]. The use of long-acting local anesthetics is advocated and it seems safe to discharge the patients before the block has worn off [86,87].

The use of regional foot blocks in conjunction with general anesthesia is thought to prolong the period of postoperative pain relief and thus be beneficial for patients undergoing day-case surgery. In one study by Clough and colleagues of outpatient bony forefoot surgery, however, supplemental foot block did not alter the consumption of postoperative analgesic tablets or overall patient satisfaction [88]. The authors concluded that although the foot block prolonged the time until postoperative pain was first perceived, it was not a major benefit when used as an analgesic in the outpatient setting.

My choice for all kinds of foot surgery (including those with an ankle tourniquet) remains the ankle block. I wash the foot and ankle and prepare a 20-ml syringe of lidocaine (15 mg/ml) and adrenaline (~7 µg/ml), and a 25 G needle. First I aim for paresthesia down in the foot by positioning the needle right behind the artery posterior to the medial malleolus, and inject 5–7 ml. Then I inject a further 5 ml in the groove lateral to the extensor tendon of the big toe in the ankle joint. From the same position I then make a fan of subcutaneous injections of 5–7 ml in the direction of the lateral malleolus and then reposition the needle to infiltrate further and back to the medial malleolus.

For unilateral knee surgery I still opt for a spinal or request the surgeon to provide appropriate cover with local anesthetic combined with using general anesthesia.

Upper limb surgery

For surgery below the elbow the axillary plexus technique is the most popular approach. Using a peripheral nerve stimulator, the humeral approach seems as reliable as the axillary approach [89]. Both techniques involve stimulation and injections into three to four sites. The lateral infra-clavicular plexus block is simpler, with only one stimulation and injection necessary to provide good blockade of all the nerves (i.e., ulnar, radial, median, and musculocutaneous nerves), as shown by Deleuze et al. [90]. It remains unclear whether the co-administration of adjuvants such as an opioid, an α_2-agonist, or ketamine is beneficial. The addition of 0.3 mg buprenorphine to the local anesthetic tripled the postoperative analgesia period in a study of axillary blocks [91]. Further studies are needed to elucidate this controversial topic. The question of dosage and volume is another interesting area of investigations. Does the same dosage diluted in a higher volume increase success rate, the area of blockage, or the duration of block? Krenn et al. compared axillary blocks with 150 mg ropivacaine diluted to 30, 40, or 60 ml and found that increasing the volume to 60 ml reduced the time to onset of motor but not sensory block [92]. No differences were found in the duration of the blocks. Although they conclude that the sensory block is the most important for a successful surgical outcome, a faster onset of motor block may be of benefit in order to determine whether it is effective.

A rapidly emerging area of interest is the use of ultrasound-guided blocks. Ultrasound in skilled hands enables the imaging of peripheral nerves and vessels and the possibility of guiding the block needle with real-time imaging, thus reducing the risk of nerve damage. The ultrasound technique has been used successfully for infraclavicular blocks [93] and also has a high success rate with axillary, supraclavicular, and interscalene blocks [94,95].

My choice is to use an interscalene block for shoulder and upper arm surgery, and an axillary block for everything beneath the middle of the upper arm. I use a 50-ml syringe with lidocaine (15 mg/ml) and 7 μg/ml adrenaline, and a 10- to 20-cm catheter in order to ease needle positioning.

For the interscalene approach I position the patient supine with their head turned 20° to the contralateral side, and ask for a small head lift to locate the interscalene groove in the level lateral to the thyroid node. Using a nerve stimulator and approaching at 45° caudally, stimulate with 0.5 mA and observe for jerks below the shoulder. Then turn down to 0.2 mA and at the same time as observing for jerks slowly inject about 40 ml with frequent aspiration checks for blood.

For the axillary approach I use a 25 G Quincke needle, abduct the patient's arm at 90°, and go for the most proximal location of the artery that is palpable. I aim for the axillary artery, aspirate, and pass through (ensured when there is no bloody aspirate). Then I slowly inject 40–50 ml while I compress the artery distal to the needle. Once finished I adduct the patient's arm and compress the injection site for 3–5 min. If I create some paresthesia whilst approaching the artery, I withdraw the needle 1 mm and inject 10 ml whilst in that position before I approach the transarterial position again.

Ilioinguinal field block for inguinal hernia repair

Aasbo et al. compared preoperative inguinal field block plus perioperative sedation with general anesthesia and wound infiltration for inguinal hernia repair [96]. They found that patients anesthetized with an inguinal field block had a shorter recovery time, less pain, better mobilization, and greater satisfaction than patients who received general anesthesia and wound infiltration. These differences lasted for the whole 1-week observation period. Even though there are reports of transient femoral nerve palsy following this technique [97], the use of inguinal field block seems to be highly recommended for inguinal hernia repair in day-case surgery as an alternative to skilled surgeons doing the local anesthesia infiltration themselves.

Intravenous regional anesthesia

This is a simple method that may sometimes be used by experienced surgeons without involving the anesthesiologist. This practice may be controversial; at the very least the surgeon should have fast and adequate backup in case of cuff failure, systemic toxicity, and convulsions. The method is most reliable when carried out on the upper extremities, although anesthesia of deeper bone/joint structures may be inadequate. Also, the surgical procedure should be limited to about 1 h, because the anesthesia will wear off, tissue hypoxia will evolve, and the discomfort caused by the cuff may become significant. The method is to establish a thin iv cannula on the dorsum of the hand and then to elevate the extremity and wrap the whole arm tightly in elastic wrapping, starting with fingers, in order to "empty" out the venous blood. Then the proximal part of a double cuff is inflated to 150 mmHg above systolic blood pressure, and the wrapping is released. Then 40–50 ml of lidocaine (5 mg/ml) is injected via the iv cannula. After 5–10 min the distal part of the cuff may be filled and then the proximal part deflated, and surgery may start. The cuff should not be released before at least 20–30 min has elapsed (risk of free lidocaine and convulsions). The method is good for superficial surgery, tendon surgery, and soft tissue procedures.

Early discharge with long-acting peripheral nerve blockade: is it safe?

Whether one should discharge patients before a peripheral block has worn off is controversial. Concerns about possible nerve damage and the risk of accidental harm to an anesthetized limb remain arguments against early discharge. In a prospective study involving 2382 peripheral nerve blocks of both the upper and lower extremities with early discharge, the incidence of complications was very low, and most patients (98%) were highly satisfied with the choice of anesthesia [98]. Only 6 patients (0.25%) had a persistent paresthesia after 7 days (which later resolved) that might have been associated with the nerve block. The authors concluded that even longer-acting local anesthetics would be beneficial in order to reduce the frequent incidence of persistent pain at 7 days [98].

Conclusions

In general, loco-regional techniques are well suited for ambulatory surgery as they are associated with less postoperative nausea and pain and possibly less cognitive dysfunction.

Fast-tracking with local anesthesia and iv sedation (see Sedation) seems to be an increasingly popular alternative to general anesthesia and seems also to reduce postoperative pain and the risk of cognitive dysfunction. Early discharge with long-acting peripheral blocks appears safe, and recent data advocate the discharge of spinal anesthesia patients before voiding, provided that some important restrictions are evaluated. Epidural anesthesia looks to have a very limited role in present clinical ambulatory praxis, but there does seem to be an ongoing role for refined spinal anesthetic techniques. Avoidance of TNS by restrictions on lidocaine use and alternative use of low-dose bupivacaine, levobupivacaine, or ropivacaine are well documented, also in combination with spinal opioids.

The different techniques are being continuously refined in order to provide fast discharge-readiness, without compromising the benefit to the patient.

My conclusions, use of loco-regional techniques in clinical practice

Local infiltration

In our unit we routinely supply the surgeon with one or two (depending on the case) 20-ml syringes of bupivacaine 2.5 mg/ml or, as will be the case with more than 20 ml, levobupivacaine 2.5 mg/ml or ropivacaine 2 mg/ml. The surgeon should use an appropriate amount to infiltrate all wound structures before and during closure of the wound, independently of what kind of anesthesia has been used. This will include instillation of local anesthesia into relevant joints after orthopedic surgery. The surgeon should be encouraged to infiltrate not only the superficial wounds, but also the deeper structures and traumatized tissue.

In some cases the surgeon will also infiltrate the area preoperatively with either the same drug or lidocaine 5–10 mg/ml; for instance, in plastic surgery, oral surgery, tonsillectomy, eye surgery, and hernia surgery. This practice should be encouraged and extended.

Infiltration of local anesthetic may be the only technique used, or local anesthetic may be given but supplemented with sedation or general anesthesia. When general anesthesia is given for a procedure that may be done under local anesthesia, it is a good rule to encourage the surgeon to give preoperative local anesthesia anyway, as if the case were being done with local infiltration alone. This will frequently be the case in our eye-surgical unit, where most procedures are done under local anesthesia alone; but those being treated under general anesthesia also receive the complete local anesthetic work-up.

For major plastic surgery, for instance breast reconstruction, we use wound catheters at the skin donor site. Ropivacaine (20 ml) is repeated every 4 h after temporarily closing the wound drains for 30 min as long as the patient is in hospital [52].

Nerve blocks and regional anesthesia

My indications for nerve blocks or regional anesthesia in ambulatory care are: (1) as a routine for cases with anticipated postoperative pain problems or (2) in individual patients who have some contraindications or there are concerns about general anesthesia with or without local anesthesia adjunct.

Orthopedic ambulatory surgery generally comes with a high expectation of postoperative pain. This does not include diagnostic joint endoscopies or endoscopies for minor procedures such as meniscus extraction from the knee. These cases do very well and have a faster turnover and more rapid recovery by using general anesthesia and local wound infiltration plus instillation into the joint. But in cases of bone surgery, osteotomies, cruciate ligament repair, and other cases of major orthopedic trauma, a regional block will usually be done, supplemented with nothing, sedation, or propofol anesthesia as required. For shoulder procedures I use an interscalene block; for elbow and lower arm, the axillary block; for foot surgery, the ankle block; and for any other case below the umbilicus, a spinal.

In cases that routinely require general anesthesia, there may still be special indications for regional block. These include the patient with suspected airway or neck problems, fat patients, patients with severe respiratory or cardiovascular disease, and fragile, elderly patients. The patient or surgeon may also make a special request to have the surgery performed under regional anesthesia.

These cases should be evaluated individually for their anesthetic. It may sometimes be appropriate to call for an anesthesiologist from outside the unit if the particular block in question is not regularly done, and also to have the option for prolonged bed stay in the PACU if a neuraxial block is used.

Sedation

Sedation is the term used to describe a drug-induced state of calm, restfulness, or drowsiness. In more clinical terms we may attribute the sleepy and undisturbed appearance to effect components such as: anxiolysis, hypnosis, analgesia, and/or amnesia. Sedation is provided to improve perceived quality for noncomatose (i.e., those not receiving general anesthesia) patients during a variety of diagnostic or therapeutic procedures. Sedation may be used as the only measure in nonpainful cases and in those cases not readily amenable to targeted use of loco-regional anesthesia. Sedation may also be an adjunct to local infiltration anesthesia or regional anesthesia.

Usually, when we observe a patient to be sleepy and quiet during sedation, we assume that the patient is doing well. However, the history of droperidol premedication shows that this may be misleading. Sedative, high doses of droperidol were extensively used for premedication in the 1970s and 1980s, because the patients became sleepy and looked quiet and comfortable. However, a high number of patients described feeling terrible and horrified, despite their outward appearance [99].

A very important question to ask when choosing a sedative technique is what quality of drug treatment the patient needs in order to maintain their wellbeing during the procedure. The answer lies in both the patient and the nature of the procedure.

Some patients will like to be asleep, as continuous sleep will remove conscious input and the memory of anything frightening or unpleasant occurring during the procedure. A prerequisite is for the sleep to be pleasant, with no nightmares, bad dreams, or unpleasant recovery. Other patients will prefer to be awake and in control, but still want an anxiolytic to reduce their anxiety. The attitude to amnesia, that is being awake and even communicating but with no recall afterwards, is more mixed. Some patients think that this would be frightening because they want to remember and control what they said and how they behaved; others would actually like to register what is going on during the procedure, for instance by looking at the television screen during a knee arthroscopy. Others will think amnesia is good idea in order to ensure the absence of unpleasant memories afterwards. For the physician in charge, an amnesic effect may be preferable if the patient experiences unpleasant inputs, but it may be problematic if the surgeon wants to educate or inform the patient during the procedure or shortly afterwards.

A further aspect of sedation is introduced when the patient is subjected to significant nociceptive simulation or pain during the procedure. When this happens an anxiolytic or hypnotic effect may help to smooth the subjective bad experience of pain. However, the patient's problem may not resolve until so much drug is given that they approach a state of general anesthesia. In these cases the logical approach is to minimize the nociceptive input, preferably by infiltration of local anesthetics into the dedicated area for the procedure undertaken, and also by using analgesic sedation.

Sedative drug selection (see also Intravenous hypnotics)

An important decision is to choose between an opioid and a hypnotic drug as the main component of sedation. Traditionally, for nonanesthesiologists the choice is between traditional opioids (e.g., morphine, oxycodone, ketobemidone, meperidine, etc.) and benzodiazepines. Access to a specific, rapidly acting antagonist (i.e., naloxone) is another safety feature of the opioids shared by the benzodiazepines (i.e., flumazenil). While these drugs are slow in onset (for both effects and side-effects), they are not safe in terms of control of breathing (especially not when combined) and they result in prolonged recovery. Thus, for the anesthesiologist it is more appropriate to use rapid and short-acting drugs, such as propofol or remifentanil. In a study comparing these drugs Servin and coworkers confirmed the expected effects of these two drug classes: remifentanil sedation resulted in more nausea and vomiting, more respiratory depression but more rapid emergence than propofol. Propofol was more reliable in terms of producing amnesia [100]. In a double-blind study, propofol or remifentanil was titrated and the observer noted equal degrees of sleepiness during ongoing leg surgery or arm surgery with loco-regional anesthetic blocks. Interestingly, but predictably, those patients sedated with remifentanil whose block was not perfect or complete reported pain significantly less frequently than did those sedated with propofol [101]. In another study Smith and coworkers found increased respiratory depression with remifentanil sedation during breast biopsy procedures done under local anesthesia when compared with propofol [102]. Thus, opioids are strongly analgesic and have some hypnotic effect as well. The anxiolytic and amnesic effects of the opioids are more controversial and inconsistent. It seems that some patients will experience these effects, whereas others do not, even with high doses. Some patients describe the opioid effect as unpleasant, in terms of increased anxiety or dysphoria [103,104]. The high frequency of nausea and vomiting may further add to the unpleasant experience of opioids. However, with a painful stimulation such as awake nasal intubation, propofol had to be dosed at a target of 3.9 µg/ml in order to have the proper effect, and at this level the patients were less responsive and cooperative (one even had a respiratory arrest) than the remifentanil patients, who managed with a target of 2.4 ng/ml [105]. This propofol dosing is higher than those levels usually considered appropriate for sedation in patients without nociceptive stimulation, who usually do well with stable plasma levels of 1–2 µg/ml propofol [100,102,106]. In a study of propofol sedation for orthopedic procedures under successful spinal anesthesia, Skipsey and colleagues were successful with a mean plasma target of 0.9 µg/ml [107]. In a study of propofol sedation during gastroscopy, a higher mean target of 2.5 µg/ml was needed [108].

To conclude, for hypnosis, anxiolysis, well maintained spontaneous breathing, amnesia, and anti-emesis, propofol is the drug of first choice. For patients in pain sedation with remifentanil is better.

Appropriate titration to effect that is timed well with nociceptive or other stimulation is a key factor of success, aiming to achieve an adequate effect without overdosing and side-effects. In their daily work, many anesthesiologists use combinations of drugs, for instance opioids together with a benzodiazepine or propofol. It should be noted though that combinations with opioids are generally synergistic in their respiratory depressive actions [109].

A new and interesting addition to our toolbox for sedation, although yet to be approved in Europe, is dexmedetomidine , which has minimal respiratory depression and preserves the pattern of natural sleep [110]. Dexmedetomidine has been used successfully for sedation in children, whereas its role in adult sedation needs further elucidation. Although theoretically attractive it appears to have a slower onset and offset than propofol, which may mean that it is not ideal for the ambulatory setting.

Monitoring needed

Basic monitoring is appropriate for routine cases, including continuous ECG, pulse oximetry, noninvasive blood pressure readings, and basic respiratory monitoring with capnography, oxygen tension, and inhalational agent concentration if these are in use. As routine patients tend to be young or middle-aged with adequate cardiovascular function and there is only a very small risk of sudden, major bleeding, an arterial line is rarely used in ambulatory surgery. However, it may be useful for checking blood gas values during pneumoperitoneum and also for controlling the rapid shifts in blood pressure that may occur during induction and positioning of patients for major procedures.

Usually one good venous line will do during induction of anesthesia. When total intravenous anesthesia (TIVA) is used, supplementation with a second iv line may be recommended for more extensive cases – one for the infusion of drugs with an ongoing Ringer's acetate solution running and the other with a slowly running colloid or crystalloid solution with the option of a rapid rate increase to control hemodynamics. It is very important to maintain visibility of the drug infusion line and also to fit one-way valves and active obstruction alarms on to the drug pumps so as to ensure that iv drugs are delivered to the patient's circulation.

As a typical ambulatory procedure rarely lasts more than 2–3 h, no major fluid shifts are involved, and with the rapid recovery no urinary catheter is needed in routine cases. A central venous line is very rarely used for similar reasons. These patients will drink and ambulate within a few hours.

The bispectral index (BIS) is the best documented mode of monitoring anesthetic depth, and is a useful, although not mandatory, adjunct. BIS is useful both for avoiding awareness if neuromuscular blockers are used [111] and for titration of the anesthetic depth for rapid emergence [112]. Overdosing of an anesthetic drug is less prone to happen when this device is used. The cost of electrodes for BIS is quite significant and there may be an option to purchase less expensive alternatives to BIS in the future, although they need to be better documented.

When neuromuscular blocking agents are used, monitoring of function is recommended, for instance by the train of four (TOF) ratio.

As with all anesthetic cases, the need for more extensive monitoring of the patient's respiratory function or hemodynamics may arise if the patient has any malfunction or serious concomitant disease or if a specific high-risk surgical procedure is being performed.

How to make a final choice of technique in the individual case?

There is no conclusive evidence to highlight any technique as being superior in terms of safety, i.e., a close to zero incidence of mortality or permanent disability. The choice must be made according to total quality for the patient and their experience as well as the cost-effectiveness for the unit. Quality for individual patients varies and depends upon personal preferences, such as being awake, fear of needles, risk, and tolerance of side-effects such as postoperative nausea and pain. Cost-effectiveness will also vary with the surgical unit in question: acquisition costs of drugs, staffing, out-of-theater induction or regional block facilities, postoperative recovery facilities, and so on. However, the following are some general approaches that reflect my personal preferences in my setting:

1. For superficial surgery or cases with minor surgical invasiveness local anesthesia with individually tailored and minimized sedation may be preferred.

2. For surgery of middling duration, in areas suitable for regional anesthesia, with an anticipated medium or high intensity of postoperative pain, a regional nerve block or centro-axial block may be recommended. The same may be valid for patients with a definite preference for regional techniques or for patients with a high risk of nausea or vomiting.

3. For other procedures general anesthesia is usually chosen, mostly due to the decreased time required for preparation and the ease of administration. With general anesthesia care must be taken to ensure optimal prophylaxis against pain and nausea in the postoperative period.

Special patients

This section must be read in conjunction with Chapter 3, where patient selection and planning are discussed. Thus for the discussion here we assume that the patient has been properly selected and prepared for ambulatory care. There will be cases that would normally necessitate inpatient status, but where you decide to give it a try as an ambulatory procedure because unplanned admission is fairly easy to accomplish if needed in your work setting. There may also be patients whose health and situation change, mandating a re-evaluation of the plan for ambulatory surgery.

The anesthetic management of such special patients should be the same in the ambulatory setting as in the inpatient setting, and is discussed extensively in major textbooks and reviews elsewhere.

Children (see also recipe in Chapter 7)

Anesthetic care of children should include the application of local anesthesia pads to both hands (i.e., EMLA® cream) to ensure painless venous access. If the child accepts oral tablets or linctus, it may be good to give an appropriate dose of paracetamol and NSAID orally 1 h or more before surgery for pain prophylaxis. If there is a problem of acceptance, there is no need to have a confrontation, as these drugs may be given iv or rectally after the start of anesthesia. Usually sedative premedication is not needed in a well-reassured child accompanied by a close relative. Use of preoperative sedatives may prolong their postoperative recovery and discharge, and also disturb their normal diurnal sleep pattern more than necessary. Nevertheless, in the very agitated child, midazolam oral mixture 0.5 mg/kg may be a good option to control the preoperative situation when needed. An alternative may be rectal diazepam suspension, 0.5–1.0 mg/kg.

A quiet and familiar atmosphere is very conducive to an uneventful preparation. Free fluid (except milk products) until 2 h before the start of anesthesia is good for the patient's mood, and if surgery is planned after lunch an early morning light breakfast (6 h in advance rule) may be very good. The child's wait in the unit should be as short as possible, and preferably their parents should be there too in a room with toys, books or a video screen. Ideally the unit should be styled with everyday furniture (so that it does not look like a hospital) and the child should not mix with discharge-ready children unless they are really happy and fully recovered.

My favorite technique for routine induction is to keep the child as normally dressed as possible (including shoes), sitting on their parent's knee with some toys available, and/or a computer screen with cartoons running close by. I prefer to use iv induction because it is safe and fast, unless you miss the vein or have to struggle vigorously. The safety concerns are potential laryngospasm, bradycardia, and also aspiration. Even though ambulatory children are required to be elective and fasting, they do occasionally have some stomach content (they fool their parents and eat or their parents do not tell you for fear of cancellation). If possible remove the EMLA patch some minutes beforehand (less skin pallor and vasoconstriction), but this is not critical. I usually show the child that the topical anesthesia works by gently squeezing their skin (do it very gently but say that you are squeezing hard!). Allow time for the vein tourniquet to take effect and flick the veins to make them stand out. After cannulation I start the Ringer's solution running and put on the pulse oximeter. Then I induce anesthesia with opioid + propofol.

As an alternative I may use inhalational induction (sevoflurane 8% in oxygen until they are deeply asleep, then obtain venous access) in the following circumstances:

- When a child or parent insists (i.e., do not change their mind in spite of gentle persuasion, for instance due to previous good experience) on inhalational induction.
- When cannulation in the EMLA-treated area looks hopeless and no good veins outside the EMLA area are visible.
- If two attempts inside the EMLA-treated area or one attempt outside the EMLA-treated area are missed.

In children who have not had EMLA or whose EMLA patch was misplaced outside a vein area, I usually make one quick attempt if there is a good vein available. I will tell the child just before skin penetration that this will hurt, but very briefly, and then the pain will stop.

For very short-lasting procedures (5–10 min) I use an oral mask, otherwise a laryngeal mask. For tonsillectomies, adenoidectomies, and dental surgery I will intubate, mostly because the surgeon is working in the mouth and may dislodge an LMA more easily than a tube, but also (in the case of tonsillectomy) to have better control of the airway in case there is profuse bleeding. This view may be challenged; with an experienced surgeon and good communication with him/her, many experienced anesthesiologists also use the LMA for adenotonsillectomies.

As to propofol pharmacology, children need about 50–100% more than adults during induction, and 25–50% more during maintenance, mostly for pharmacokinetic reasons (larger initial distribution volume and higher clearance, see Chapter 4). For opioids and muscle relaxants the dose will be about the same (per kg) as in adults, although a little more remifentanil may be needed due to its higher clearance.

For volatiles the MAC values are 25–50% higher (depending on age, see Chapter 4) than in adults. If nitrous oxide is readily available I still think it is a useful adjunct, 50% (small children) to 66% in oxygen, in addition to either iv or inhalational anesthesia. Nitrous oxide is not a cardiorespiratory depressant in healthy outpatients, has a very rapid on–off effect, and will reduce the required dose of other, slower, agents. When using nitrous oxide care should be taken to ensure that, at the end of the case, there is adequate ventilation on oxygen-enriched gas after turning the nitrous oxide off. Because much nitrous oxide is released into the lungs during the first 3–5 min after cessation, a combination of hypoventilation and just giving air may result in hypoxia. A pulse oximeter should always be used, and will reveal (although a little delayed) if any hypoxia is emerging.

Sevoflurane is definitely the gas of choice for induction of inhalational anesthesia, and may very well be used for maintenance, perhaps combined with an opioid. However, sevoflurane is associated with a high incidence (up to 10–20%) of severe, short-lasting agitation during emergence [113]. The incidence will be lower when the child emerges with their parents close by and has received adequate analgesia (local anesthetic and/or opioids), but is still bothersome in some patients. The incidence is lower with desflurane emergence and even lower, in fact barely noticeable, with propofol [114]. Desflurane is not suitable for inhalational induction (bad smell, irritation, laryngospasm), however it may be an alternative for maintenance after sevoflurane induction, because it causes less postoperative agitation, has a slightly faster emergence and causes less respiratory depression [115]. Another alternative is to use a small bolus dose or a short-lasting infusion of propofol at the end of the case to avoid emergence agitation and also to provide some short-lasting anti-emetic effect.

As with all patients, the surgeon should be encouraged to use local anesthesia as extensively as possible for postoperative pain relief, and the anesthesiologist may also use a sacral block with 0.5–1.0 ml bupivacaine (2.5 mg/ml) in appropriate patients (i.e., hernia, perineal surgery, external genitalia, testicular retention, etc.). Further, non-opioids including NSAIDs may be used, perhaps dexamethasone for both pain and emesis prophylaxis. The new cyclooxygenase II (COX-II) inhibitors are not yet approved for children, due to a lack of studies and documentation, but will probably evolve as alternatives, especially in cases where traditional NSAIDs are contraindicated.

The elderly

The elderly are generally well suited for ambulatory surgery and will profit and appreciate ambulatory care if it is otherwise compatible with safety and quality. The elderly generally have a lower risk for PONV and a higher pain threshold than younger patients. However, once their threshold for pain is reached, the elderly often have a low tolerance for pain when present. Although general anesthetic routines may be applied and concomitant disease should be treated as usual, the anesthetic management of even healthy elderly patients needs some adjustment. The microcirculation in the brain and muscles slows down with age, thus the wash-in and wash-out of drugs (hypnotics, opioids, relaxants, inhalational agents) is also slowed down and the onset–offset of effect slower. The elderly have a stiffer cardiovascular system and often a higher systolic blood pressure, but are more prone to hypotension during induction than younger adults. The maximum effect on respiration and especially blood pressure after induction is quite delayed compared with how quickly they fall asleep, and for that reason a slow titration of induction drug is recommended, with a rapid and smooth setup for assisted ventilation and gentle vasopressor use. Titration is important, also because the inter-individual difference in response to standard doses is high in the elderly.

With propofol, a 25–50% reduction in induction dose is recommended due to pharmacokinetics, as the elderly have a small initial distribution volume (V1; see Chapter 4). Whether the elderly have increased sensitivity to hypnotic agents is disputed, but this is probably present to some degree, necessitating a slightly lower dosing level or target during maintenance. Clearance is fairly unchanged, thus when the proper target is reached, the elderly will require the same maintenance as younger patients.

With the opioids the story is different. Generally the pharmacokinetics and plasma concentrations are quite similar to those in younger patients, but the sensitivity to opioids is increased and almost doubled in a patient of 70–80 years compared with in the young. For this reason both induction and opioid maintenance should be reduced by 50–100% in the elderly. For inhalational agents MAC is less and subsequently there is a reduced need of 10–30% in the elderly, whereas the dosing of neuromuscular blockers will be quite similar to that for young patients.

As with all fragile patients, loco-regional techniques should be encouraged in the elderly, although there are no good studies showing their superiority in terms of safety or mortality in ambulatory or minor/intermediately invasive surgery. Nevertheless, loco-regional techniques are beneficial in the elderly with pulmonary or airway problems, but care should be taken to avoid severe hypotension during spinal anesthesia in the fragile elderly patient.

The ASA III pulmonary/airway disease patient

In patients with asthma and some patients with chronic obstructive pulmonary disease (COPD) preoperative inhalation of aerosol is indicated if this treatment is available. Loco-regional techniques or general anesthesia techniques that allow for spontaneous ventilation may be preferred if the pulmonary function is very reduced. If the patient needs to be ventilated, controlled ventilation with positive end-expiratory pressure (PEEP) and pressure-controlled mode may be best for lung physiology. If neuromuscular agents are used, proper reversal is very important; such patients should definitely be monitored with a TOF guard and there may be a rare indication for sugammadex in order to make the reversal rapid and complete, i.e., a TOF ratio of at least 0.9.

When pulmonary patients are sedated, oxygen supplements should be closely titrated and only given when indicated. In such cases capnography or other means of respiration monitoring should be added to the pulse oximeter.

Patients with sleep apnea syndrome (SAS), if eligible for ambulatory care (see Chapter 3), should, if possible, be treated with a loco-regional technique. If deep sedation or general anesthesia is needed, long-lasting opioids should be avoided or minimized through the use of an optimal non-opioid analgesia regimen. A continuous positive airways pressure (CPAP) mask may be used in the PACU if the patient is very sleepy, and if the patient is used to CPAP he or she should be urged to use it the first few nights home after surgery. If the patient is in need of CPAP, but not used to it previously, he or she should be referred for overnight stay with continuous monitoring.

The cardiovascular disease patient

Hypertension

Occasionally patients present with a high blood pressure (i.e., above 180/110 mmHg) reading, with or without a previous history of hypertension or treatment, for their first preoperative evaluation on the day of surgery. Usually this is not a reason to cancel unless the pressure is very high (above 200/120 mmHg) or there are clinical symptoms (headache, heart murmurs). The threshold for cancellation may also have to do with type of surgery and anesthesia planned.

If one proceeds with the case after a high reading, the measurement should be repeated many times during reassuring discussions and preparation, as anxiety may be an important enhancer of blood pressure. One could also test a very small dose of midazolam (1–2 mg) or propofol (20–40 mg) for anxiolysis to see if the pressure normalizes. If blood pressure remains high it may be necessary to give a beta-blocker, for instance metoprolol 1 mg iv repeated and titrated every 2–3 min until the blood pressure values are reasonable. It is also important to be careful and to avoid adding epinephrine to any local anesthesia in such cases.

Angina pectoris

It is important that these patients are in a stable phase and receive their regular treatment and prophylaxis. It is especially important that they receive their regular beta-blockers and cholesterol-reducing agents (statins), as a peroperative break in medication may increase the risk of arrhythmia and infarction. If they can be managed with a loco-regional technique (be careful with or avoid adrenaline adjuvant!), being awake or sedated will increase the chances of discovering signs of angina. These patients should be on oxygen (2 l/min by nasal cannula) and be monitored with a precordial ECG with the ST segment clearly visible for evaluation. The aim is for stable hemodynamics, avoiding hypertension and particularly tachycardia (anything above 100–110 beats /min). Hypotension and bradycardia may also be dangerous. Should angina or ST depression occur during the procedure, nasal or iv nitro-glycerine and 100% oxygen ventilation should be tried, and the procedure terminated.

Previous coronary infarction

Patients who have had an infarction should be treated as angina patients (see above), perhaps with extra measures if they have concomitant heart failure or are on antithrombotic treatment (see later).

Heart failure

The treatment of these patients should focus on the underlying cause of heart failure. They will benefit from continuous perioperative use of all their basic cardiovascular medications (except perhaps anticoagulants, see Chapter 3). Efforts should be made to keep them normovolemic, as both hypervolemia and hypovolemia may create problems. They will benefit from anesthetic management that allows spontaneous ventilation if possible. Laying the patients with their upper body slightly elevated also improves their function unless they are hypovolemic or become hypotensive under such conditions.

Heart valve dysfunction

Patients with aortic or mitral insufficiency may be treated according to any symptoms they have of concomitant heart failure or angina. For patients with aortic or mitral stenosis who are acceptable for ambulatory surgery, care should be taken to avoid tachycardia or any tachyarrhythmia. Hypovolemia should be avoided, and for aortic stenosis patients care should be taken to avoid strong peripheral vasodilatation, as with spinal or epidural blocks.

Pacemaker or intracardiac defibrillator (ICD)

It is best to avoid electrocauterization in such patients, but bipolar technology is well accepted when needed. If a unipolar technique is needed, care should be taken to place the electrodes and circuit as far as possible away from the heart region. Short intermittent pulses of cauterization are less risky than prolonged continuous use. Some pacemakers may be programmed at a fixed rate during surgery if needed, and almost all pacemakers will operate at a fixed rate if a strong, specialized magnet is placed on the skin surface. A magnet will usually block an ICD device, which may be useful in some situations with electrocautery near the heart. In this case an external defibrillator should be immediately available, just in case magnet removal does not immediately solve a need for defibrillation during surgery.

Anticoagulated patients
See Chapter 3.

The obese patient [116, 117] (see also recipe in Chapter 7)
These patients are prone to concomitant health problems (see Chapter 3), which should be dealt with accordingly.

Advice and measures to take in advance
As with all patients, cessation of smoking 4–5 weeks before scheduled surgery improves respiratory function, and this is especially valuable in the obese because they are more prone to airway problems than others. Stopping 1–3 weeks before surgery, if the patient is a daily smoker, is not advised as airway reactivity and secretions may be temporarily increased for some weeks after smoking is stopped. Nevertheless, the regular smoker should be strongly advised not to smoke on the day of surgery, as even a single cigarette will result in some carboxyhemoglobin formation, which will reduce the oxygen-binding capacity of blood for some hours afterwards.

Especially when intra-abdominal procedures (laparoscopy, laparotomy) are planned, it is a good safety measure to advise the patient to reduce, even minimally, their weight in the weeks ahead of surgery, by adopting a high-protein, low-carbohydrate diet. This is because most obese people have an enlarged and fragile fatty liver. By diet and weight reduction for a period of weeks the liver shrinks and becomes less fragile. This is important as it facilitates surgical access to the abdomen and reduces the risk of liver tear or bleeding.

Gastroesophageal reflux disease occurs in about 20–30% of obese patients, and they may be at risk for perioperative regurgitation of stomach acid into the airways. A good way of reducing both the amount and acidity of the gastric contents is to use a proton pump inhibitor (e.g., omeprazole). The first dose should be taken at least a few hours before surgery, but best practice is to give it the evening before and then again on the morning of surgery. If this has not occurred, some sips of fluid antacid (sodium citrate) prior to anesthetic induction may be an alternative solution, although this is only effective on fluid pH and not volume.

In patients with suspected sleep apnea and planned general anesthesia or opioid use, the optimal strategy is to carry out overnight polysomnography well in advance of surgery, and to fit the patient with a CPAP device so that they can become familiar with using it. Patients with a CPAP device should be urged to bring it with them on the day of surgery, for use in the PACU; its use is mandatory for the first few nights at home.

In patients with respiratory problems, especially COPD, it may be useful to refer them preoperatively to a physiotherapist to clear their chest and be taught how to cough, breathe, and mobilize the lungs after surgery.

As to fasting rules, the speed of gastric emptying in obese patients is similar to that in lean patients. Thus, if no physiologic cause of gastrointestinal obstruction or slowing is evident, they should have nothing to eat (including milk) for the 6 hours before surgery and no clear fluids in the last 2 hours. Some preoperative tablets may be allowed to be taken with a few sips of water up to 1 hour ahead of anesthetic induction.

Premedication

Due to the increased incidence and risk of airway obstruction in obese patients, they should generally not have anxiolytic or opioid premedication. If there is a strong indication a benzodiazepine may be used, but the patients should then not be left alone, but be observed or have pulse oximetry. Establishing an iv line is safe practice, because midazolam or diazepam can then be carefully titrated and also because rapid injection of the benzodiazepine antagonist, flumazenil, is then an option if needed. Opioid premedication should only be used when needed for preoperative pain, and then in titrated doses with subsequent monitoring.

The time for premedication, one to two hours ahead of surgery, may also be a good time to give other drugs that benefit the patient: oral analgesics (paracetamol, NSAID), prophylactic antibiotics, or thrombosis prophylaxis. As obese patients have an increased propensity to thrombosis, pulmonary embolism, and wound infections, drug prophylaxis will more frequently be indicated in the obese than in the lean, but still depends upon the type of surgery.

Choice of anesthetic technique

Loco-regional anesthesia is the preferred technique for the obese. An axillary plexus approach or a spinal injection is usually possible, whereas other blocks may be more difficult with fat tissue obscuring normal anatomy. Skilled use of ultrasound technology may be a major step forward in these patients, as nerve structures may be quite clearly located within or behind fat tissue on the screen. When general anesthesia is needed or chosen, it is important for the surgeon to infiltrate the wound areas and surrounding structures with local anesthetic (LIA technique) to reduce postoperative opioid consumption. If sedation is needed for a loco-regional technique, the dose should be titrated carefully and kept to the minimum, as airway obstruction will occur much more frequently even during light sleep. If general anesthesia has to be used, spontaneous ventilation and a low or moderate duration of procedure are favored, as is anything that can minimize the need for postoperative opioids.

Issues for general anesthesia induction

Usually it will be possible to gain iv access in these patients, for instance at the inside of the lower forearm there are some thin veins not covered by fat. However, occasionally one may have to resort to ultrasound-guided access to a central vein. During induction the patients should be elevated with their trunk at 20–30° (half-sitting), preferably with the aid of a special pillow or by adjusting the operating table. This position prevents regurgitation, improves lung function (compared to when supine), and also facilitates laryngoscopy. Rapid sequence induction is not needed in these patients if they otherwise fulfill fasting criteria. Proper preoxygenation with a tight-fitting mask and a positive end-expiratory pressure (PEEP) of $10\,cmH_2O$ is very useful, and shown to result in an extra 1–2 min before desaturation if airway problems arise later on [118]. An end-tidal oxygen concentration of 80–90% on mask is a sign of successful preoxygenation. A combination of LMA and spontaneous ventilation is beneficial for airway reactivity and lung physiology especially in the obese. However, if controlled ventilation is needed, the inspiratory pressure will often be higher in the obese, especially during laparoscopies or laparotomies, which may necessitate endotracheal intubation. After intubation, a recruitment maneuver is beneficial to inflate the lungs, and then maintain PEEP at $10\,cmH_2O$ throughout the case, and repeat the recruitment maneuver before extubation. Pressure-control ventilation mode is better for lung physiology, whereas the volume mode is safer in terms of delivering an appropriate tidal volume (which should be adjusted to ideal weight), especially during gastric surgery where the high peritoneal pressure may result in very low tidal volumes with the non-adjusted pressure-control mode.

Issues during maintenance

All fat-soluble agents are problematic to dose in the obese, because they distribute according to slightly more than the ideal weight initially (i.e., corrected ideal body weight), and then increasingly to the total weight as the fat is steadily loaded with the drug. An exception is remifentanil, which is degraded before reaching the fat, and thus is very suitable for continued use in the obese. Propofol may be used for induction according to corrected ideal body weight, but maintenance beyond 30–60 min calls for an increase in dose, which is best titrated with the aid of a brain function monitor, such as BIS. Among inhalational agents, desflurane is the best in terms of less tissue binding and more rapid emergence compared with other inhalational agents [119], except nitrous oxide.

Emergence and postoperative issues

With careful use of maintenance drugs, it should be possible to have a rapid emergence and extubation in obese ambulatory cases. It is very important to be generous with anti-emetic prophylaxis in these patients and to provide optimal nonopioid analgesia. In the PACU, the half-sitting position and rapid mobilization should be encouraged.

Diabetes mellitus

General advice to these patients is to behave completely as normal on the day before surgery: ordinary food, ordinary dosing of antidiabetics, including insulin. No food or antidiabetics should be taken after midnight before the day of admission. Patients should then be admitted to the unit on the morning of surgery for blood glucose testing and subsequent surgery early in the day. If the blood sugar is above 10 mmol/l it is appropriate to start an insulin infusion of 2–4 units per hour and then check the blood sugar every hour when the patient is awake and every 30 min if the patient is asleep or under general anesthesia. With values between 5 and 10 mmol/l no insulin or sugar should be given, just check every 1–2 h while the patient is in the unit and more frequently during sleep or general anesthesia. Repeated control of blood sugar levels to within a range of 5–10 mmol/l is only needed for those patients on insulin or oral antidiabetics, as there is a small risk of declining blood sugar due to the residual effect of antidiabetics taken the previous day. With values below 5 mmol/l a 5% glucose infusion (50 mg/ml) should be given at a rate of 50–100 ml/h, according to blood sugar values (see above). With values of less than 3 mmol/l an immediate bolus of 20 ml concentrated glucose should be given first and no anesthesia or sedation should be started until values are above 5 mmol/l.

Alcohol or drug abuse

If a patient is obviously drugged or drunk, or if they show overt signs of withdrawal, the case should be canceled. Otherwise, with these patients one should be prepared for their increased need for centrally acting drugs. A loco-regional technique is preferable but regardless of the method chosen optimal nonopioid pain prophylaxis and treatment should be instituted and continued postoperatively. For patients on regular methadone, buprenorphine, or other opioids (including chronic pain patients) the general rule is to have them continue with their ordinary drug regimen throughout the perioperative course and to add propofol, inhalational agents, and perhaps remifentanil for general anesthesia.

If additional opioid is needed in the immediate postoperative phase despite optimal nonopioid treatment (including local anesthesia infiltration), they should be given titrated doses of fentanyl or another pure opioid agonist.

In such patients one should always be prepared for unexpected admission and remain highly alert to the possibility that it may not be safe to send them home for further analgesic treatment and surveillance of complications.

Psychiatric patients, patients with cognitive dysfunction or disabilities

These patients will usually benefit from their stay in the hospital environment being as short and uneventful as possible. Helpful steps to take are: having a known chaperone stay with them until they are asleep, not waiting for too long in the unit, staying in a quiet and friendly area before surgery, avoiding any unnecessary changes in clothing, having a sedative tablet beforehand, and having a smooth and uneventful induction. The latter should be individually tailored; most do best with a thin venous needle sited in an area pretreated with a local anesthesia pad, whereas others are more comfortable being induced with a gentle mask and 8% sevoflurane in oxygen.

The use of psychopharmaceuticals may interfere with the dosing of general anesthetics. Although TIVA with propofol and remifentanil is well suited for short procedures in these patients, a more rapid and clearheaded recovery is seen with desflurane maintenance, which may be the method of choice for any procedure lasting more than 1–2 h.

Acute disease

Such patients are occasionally accepted for ambulatory care. When treating such patients, one should be aware of pain issues and of preoperative use of opioids, which may place these patients in a nonfasting status, which is otherwise rarely seen in the ambulatory unit. Thus, such cases may call for rapid sequence induction with propofol and suxamethonium, or high-dose rocuronium, which may be reversed effectively by (quite expensive) sugammadex.

Pregnancy

In general pregnant women should be given safe, traditional anesthetic drugs; loco-regional techniques are preferable although general anesthesia with propofol, opioids, and inhalational agents may be used when indicated.

NSAIDS, COX-II inhibitors, glucocorticoids, and nitrous oxide should be avoided, although dangers of their short-term use are not documented.

During the last trimester, and especially for procedures in or near the abdomen/peritoneum, a consult with an obstetrician should be made in order to plan for any use of drugs to prevent the start of uterine contractions during the procedure.

Breastfeeding patients

Any anesthesia may be given and the mother may breastfeed the child as planned, even first thing postoperatively. The only precaution is to avoid large doses of benzodiazepines, codeine, or long-lasting opioids in the perioperative setting.

Other causes for not being an ASA I or II patient

Kidney disease

Urinary catheterization is usually not needed in ambulatory care and should only be done for distinct indications. This procedure always carries a risk of infection, which may be bad for some kidney disease patients. One should be careful with the dosing of drugs that are eliminated through the kidneys or have active metabolites that may accumulate: morphine, muscle relaxants (except suxamethonium, mivacurium, cisatracurium), and meperidine. Drugs that are potentially toxic to the kidney should generally be avoided, such as: NSAIDs, COX-II inhibitors, aminoglycosides, and X-ray contrast.

Liver disease

With severe liver failure some drugs will have prolonged elimination: propofol, barbiturates, most of the opioids (except remifentanil), and most of the muscle relaxants (except suxamethonium, mivacurium, cisatracurium). How toxic paracetamol is when given in severe liver failure is disputed; the best solution is probably to avoid paracetamol, or dose carefully (half dose), and only for a few days at most.

Gastric tubing may be dangerous in patients with esophageal varices and is best avoided where there is doubt.

Thyroid disorders

A low or high metabolism may interfere with the dosing requirements of general anesthetics, but usually not to any great extent if the condition is well regulated in advance.

In cases of overt goiter, airway management may be problematic, and one should prepare for fiberoptic intubation in case such problems arise.

As always with airway risk management, goiter may be a strong indication for loco-regional techniques and spontaneous breathing.

Rheumatoid arthritis, ankylosing spondylitis (Bechterew disease), other rheumatic conditions

The main concern here for patients is handling of the neck and its implications for airway management; therefore, loco-regional anesthesia is the preferred technique. The patients should always be asked to perform a maximal mouth opening and maximal neck extension before sleep is induced. If range of movement is poor one should discuss the case and perhaps arrange to have extra resources available, or consider an awake fiberoptic nasal intubation for those rare cases where an LMA cannot pass through the mouth. Otherwise, it may be wise to position the patient's head optimally for LMA or facial mask management before inducing sleep, and to maintain this position throughout the procedure by supporting pillows. Muscle relaxation is good to avoid if possible because muscular tension will protect the patient from inadvertent gross movements of the neck.

Neurologic diseases

Myasthenic patients should take their ordinary medication; muscle relaxants and benzodiazepines should be avoided. If neuromuscular block is needed, very small (10–20% of normal) and titrated doses should be used, and rocuronium with sugammadex reversal may be strongly indicated in order to avoid interference with the cholinergic balance.

Epileptic patients

These patients should take their ordinary medication; it may be wise to reinforce them with a small dose of midazolam before the start of anesthesia in severe cases. Otherwise, they may have an anesthetic as usual, although concern over high-dose (>1 MAC) sevoflurane has been raised as this drug may cause epileptogenic activity on electroencephalography (EEG).

Allergy

In the multi-allergic patient it may be wise to give histamine type 1 and type 2 antagonists beforehand (e.g., promethazine + ranitidine) as well as glucocorticoid slowly during induction. Be careful to avoid placing the patient in contact with latex and only give nonallergenic drugs, such as inhalational agents and synthetic opioids. Propofol or barbiturates may be used for induction, but if in doubt or in cases of severe multi-allergy midazolam or ketamine may be safer; sevoflurane induction is optimal in this regard.

Problems with previous anesthesia or with anesthesia in close family

In patients with previous unexplained jaundice (inhalational hepatitis?), inhalational agents may be best avoided; with cholinesterase deficiencies, suxamethonium and mivacurium should be avoided.

If malignant hyperthermia is suspected in the patient or their close family, have a low threshold for using only safe drugs such as propofol, barbiturates, opioids, ketamine, and nondepolarizing relaxants. A clean anesthesia system with no traces of inhalational agents should be used. Patients with a strong suspicion in the history should be observed for a few hours in the unit, as even small traces of inhalational agents or suxamethonium in the perioperative environment may induce malignant hyperthermia, which may start in the postoperative phase.

Preoperative medication (see also Chapter 3)

Consider starting or reinforcing the following drugs perioperatively.

Anticoagulation [120]

There is much debate about, and little evidence in the literature for, the use of extra anticoagulation for selected patients or procedures in ambulatory surgery. Most hematologists claim that, in order to be better than placebo, patients should have daily injections for at least 7–10 days after the procedure. With a minor ambulatory surgical procedure, patient motivation for, and compliance with, these injections may be hard to gain over a period of many days once they are fully fit and otherwise back to normal. For this reason, most ambulatory units do not practice routine anticoagulation for any group of patients, just for those who have a specific indication. This may include prolonged surgery with much trauma and immobilization afterwards, procedures that are rare in ambulatory care. Another high-risk group seems to be those having knee and lower limb surgery during which a tourniquet is applied for more than 60 min.

As to patient risk factors they include: obesity, smoking, oral contraceptive use, steroid use, deep venous thrombosis, or lung emboli in their own or close-family history, pregnancy or being in the postpartum period.

When two or more of these factors are present it may be justified to initiate thrombosis prophylaxis. The indication is also strong for patients with an own or family history of thrombosis, and in those with Leiden factor mutations. In those cases it is helpful to have a hematological consult before the procedure, especially for Leiden patients, some of whom have a high risk while others do not. The indication for anticoagulation is less for short-lasting procedures with minor tissue trauma and rapid mobilization afterwards.

Prophylaxis should be started with the first dose given 2–4 h after surgery (when hemostasis is assured) and then preferably continued for 7–10 days with dalteparin 5000 units or enoxaparin 40 mg or an equivalent of another drug. A more simplified, although not documented, approach in patients with a moderately increased risk is to give an injection of anticoagulant (see above) in the unit and then use a platelet-inhibiting COX-I-predominant NSAID (e.g., naproxen) as combined painkiller and antithrombotic during the first week after surgery.

Patients using glucocorticoids

A well-known rule in anesthesia is to have patients using glucocorticoids regularly (anything more than 5 mg prednisolone daily or equivalent) receive a booster dose of glucocorticoid to mimic the physiological stress response during surgery, as their adrenal cortex is not normally responsive. Although the usefulness for major trauma and disease is well documented for this practice, this is not the case for minor or intermediate procedures such as most cases in ambulatory surgery. However, as glucocorticoids are good for both anti-emesis and analgesia in almost any surgical patient, it may be a good rule to give all these patients a standard adult dose of 8 mg dexamethasone (or equivalent) during the procedure. The effect will last for 2–3 days, and after that they are covered by their usual medication.

References

1. White PF, Eng M. Fast-track anesthetic techniques for ambulatory surgery. *Curr Opin Anaesthesiol* 2007;**20**:545–57.

2. Raeder JC. Total intravenous anaesthesia – free from nitrous oxide, free from problems? *Acta Anaesthesiol Scand* 1994;**38**:769–70.

3. Sarkela MO, Ermes MJ, van Gils MJ, et al. Quantification of epileptiform electroencephalographic activity during sevoflurane mask induction. *Anesthesiology* 2007;**107**:928–38.

4. Beskow A, Westrin P. Sevoflurane causes more postoperative agitation in children than does halothane. *Acta Anaesthesiol Scand* 1999;**43**:536–41.

5. Ghatge S, Lee J, Smith I. Sevoflurane: an ideal agent for adult day-case anesthesia? *Acta Anaesthesiol Scand* 2003;**47**:917–31.

6. Raeder J, Kvande G, Dale O, Breivik H. [Postoperative liver damage due to halothane. Should we stop using halothane for adult patients?] *Tidsskr Nor Laegeforen* 1984;**104**:2097–9.

7. Gupta A, Stierer T, Zuckerman R, et al. Comparison of recovery profile after ambulatory anesthesia with propofol, isoflurane, sevoflurane and desflurane: a systematic review. *Anesth Analg* 2004;**98**:632–41, table.

8. Gupta A. Analgesia techniques for day cases. In: Lemos P, Jarrett P, Philip B, eds. *Day Surgery – Development and Practice*, London: IAAS, 2006: 208–28.

9. Dupont J, Tavernier B, Ghosez Y, et al. Recovery after anaesthesia for pulmonary surgery: desflurane, sevoflurane and isoflurane. *Br J Anaesth* 1999;**82**:355–9.

10. Mayer J, Boldt J, Rohm KD, et al. Desflurane anesthesia after sevoflurane inhaled induction reduces severity of emergence agitation in children undergoing minor ear-nose-throat surgery compared with sevoflurane induction and maintenance. *Anesth Analg* 2006;**102**:400–4.

11. Holm EP, Sessler DI, Standl T, am Esch JS. Shivering following normothermic desflurane or isoflurane anesthesia. *Acta Anaesthesiol Scand Suppl* 1997;**111**:321–2.

12. Apfel CC, Korttila K, Abdalla M, et al. A factorial trial of six interventions for the prevention of postoperative nausea and vomiting. *N Engl J Med* 2004;**350**:2441–51.

13. Hedelin H, Holmang S, Wiman L. [Outpatient treatment of bladder cancer – lower cost and satisfied patients]. *Nord Med* 1997;**112**:48–51.

14. Raeder J, Gupta A, Pedersen FM. Recovery characteristics of sevoflurane- or propofol-based anaesthesia for day-care surgery. *Acta Anaesthesiol Scand* 1997;**41**:988–94.

15. Gozdemir M, Sert H, Yilmaz N, et al. Remifentanil-propofol in vertebral disk operations: hemodynamics and recovery versus desflurane-N(2)O inhalation anesthesia. *Adv Ther* 2007;**24**:622–31.

16. Rohm KD, Riechmann J, Boldt J, et al. Total intravenous anesthesia with propofol and remifentanil is associated with a nearly twofold higher incidence in postanesthetic shivering than desflurane-fentanyl anesthesia. *Med Sci Monit* 2006;**12**: CR452–CR456.

17. Arellano RJ, Pole ML, Rafuse SE, et al. Omission of nitrous oxide from a propofol-based anesthetic does not affect the recovery of women undergoing outpatient gynecologic surgery. *Anesthesiology* 2000;**93**:332–9.

18. Tramer M, Moore A, McQuay H. Omitting nitrous oxide in general anaesthesia: meta-analysis of intraoperative awareness and postoperative emesis in randomized controlled trials. *Br J Anaesth* 1996;**76**:186–93.

19. Hoymork SC, Raeder J, Grimsmo B, Steen PA. Bispectral index, predicted and measured drug levels of target-controlled infusions of remifentanil and propofol during laparoscopic cholecystectomy and emergence. *Acta Anaesthesiol Scand* 2000;**44**:1138–44.

20. Lehmann A, Boldt J, Thaler E, et al. Bispectral index in patients with target-controlled or manually controlled infusion of propofol. *Anesth Analg* 2002;**95**:639–44, table.

21. Guignard B, Bossard AE, Coste C, et al. Acute opioid tolerance: intraoperative remifentanil increases postoperative pain and morphine requirement. *Anesthesiology* 2000;**93**:409–17.

22. Chia YY, Liu K, Wang JJ, et al. Intraoperative high dose fentanyl induces postoperative fentanyl tolerance. *Can J Anaesth* 1999;**46**:872–7.

23. Celerier E, Rivat C, Jun Y, et al. Long-lasting hyperalgesia induced by fentanyl in rats: preventive effect of ketamine. *Anesthesiology* 2000;**92**:465–72.

24. Lenz H, Raeder J, Hoymork SC. Administration of fentanyl before remifentanil-based anaesthesia has no influence on post-operative pain or analgesic consumption. *Acta Anaesthesiol Scand* 2008;**52**:149–54.

25. Joshi GP, Inagaki Y, White PF, et al. Use of the laryngeal mask airway as an alternative to the tracheal tube during ambulatory anesthesia. *Anesth Analg* 1997;**85**:573–7.

26. Rasmussen LS, Johnson T, Kuipers HM, et al. Does anaesthesia cause postoperative cognitive dysfunction? A randomised study of regional versus general anaesthesia in 438 elderly patients. *Acta Anaesthesiol Scand* 2003;**47**:260–6.

27. Raeder J. Regional anaesthesia. In: Smith I, ed. *Day Care Anaesthesia*, London: BMJ Books, 2000: 97–126.

28. Warner MA, Shields SE, Chute CG. Major morbidity and mortality within 1 month of ambulatory surgery and anesthesia. *JAMA* 1993;**270**:1437–41.

29. Ben-David B, DeMeo PJ, Lucyk C, Solosko D. Minidose lidocaine-fentanyl spinal anesthesia in ambulatory surgery: prophylactic nalbuphine versus nalbuphine plus droperidol. *Anesth Analg* 2002;**95**:1596–600, table.

30. Bromage PR. Neurological complications of subarachnoid and epidural anaesthesia. *Acta Anaesthesiol Scand* 1997;**41**:439–44.

31. Auroy Y, Benhamou D, Bargues L, et al. Major complications of regional anesthesia in France: The SOS Regional Anesthesia Hotline Service. *Anesthesiology* 2002;**97**:1274–80.

32. Vila H, Jr., Soto R, Cantor AB, Mackey D. Comparative outcomes analysis of procedures performed in physician offices and ambulatory surgery centers. *Arch Surg* 2003;**138**:991–5.

33. Pavlin DJ, Chen C, Penaloza DA, et al. Pain as a factor complicating recovery and

discharge after ambulatory surgery. *Anesth Analg* 2002;**95**:627–34, table.

34. Dahl V, Gierloff C, Omland E, Raeder JC. Spinal, epidural or propofol anaesthesia for out-patient knee arthroscopy? *Acta Anaesthesiol Scand* 1997;**41**:1341–5.

35. Borgeat A, Ekatodramis G, Schenker CA. Postoperative nausea and vomiting in regional anesthesia: a review. *Anesthesiology* 2003;**98**:530–47.

36. Moller JT, Cluitmans P, Rasmussen LS, et al. Long-term postoperative cognitive dysfunction in the elderly ISPOCD1 study. ISPOCD investigators. International Study of Post-Operative Cognitive Dysfunction. *Lancet* 1998;**351**:857–61.

37. Rasmussen LS, Johnson T, Kuipers HM, et al. Does anaesthesia cause postoperative cognitive dysfunction? A randomised study of regional versus general anaesthesia in 438 elderly patients. *Acta Anaesthesiol Scand* 2003;**47**:260–6.

38. Servin FS, Raeder JC, Merle JC, et al. Remifentanil sedation compared with propofol during regional anaesthesia. *Acta Anaesthesiol Scand* 2002;**46**:309–15.

39. Cravero JP. Risk and safety of pediatric sedation/anesthesia for procedures outside the operating room. *Curr Opin Anaesthesiol* 2009;**22**:509–13.

40. Zeyneloglu P, Pirat A, Candan S, et al. Dexmedetomidine causes prolonged recovery when compared with midazolam/fentanyl combination in outpatient shock wave lithotripsy. *Eur J Anaesthesiol* 2008;**25**:961–7.

41. Watkins AC, White PF. Fast-tracking after ambulatory surgery. *J Perianesth Nurs* 2001;**16**:379–87.

42. Apfelbaum JL, Walawander CA, Grasela TH, et al. Eliminating intensive postoperative care in same-day surgery patients using short-acting anesthetics. *Anesthesiology* 2002;**97**:66–74.

43. Payne K, Moore EW, Elliott RA, et al. Anaesthesia for day case surgery: a survey of paediatric clinical practice in the UK. *Eur J Anaesthesiol* 2003;**20**:325–30.

44. Lennox PH, Chilvers C, Vaghadia H. Selective spinal anesthesia versus desflurane anesthesia in short duration outpatient gynecological laparoscopy: a pharmacoeconomic comparison. *Anesth Analg* 2002;**94**:565–8.

45. Danelli G, Berti M, Casati A, et al. Spinal block or total intravenous anaesthesia with propofol and remifentanil for gynaecological outpatient procedures. *Eur J Anaesthesiol* 2002;**19**:594–9.

46. Li S, Coloma M, White PF, et al. Comparison of the costs and recovery profiles of three anesthetic techniques for ambulatory anorectal surgery. *Anesthesiology* 2000;**93**:1225–30.

47. Panni M, Segal S. New local anesthetics. Are they worth the cost? *Anesthesiol Clin North America* 2003;**21**:19–38.

48. Aasvang EK, Hansen JB, Malmstrom J, et al. The effect of wound instillation of a novel purified capsaicin formulation on postherniotomy pain: a double-blind, randomized, placebo-controlled study. *Anesth Analg* 2008;**107**:282–91.

49. Klaastad O, Smedby O, Thompson GE, et al. Distribution of local anesthetic in axillary brachial plexus block: a clinical and magnetic resonance imaging study. *Anesthesiology* 2002;**96**:1315–24.

50. Rawal N. Incisional and intra-articular infusions. *Best Pract Res Clin Anaesthesiol* 2002;**16**:321–43.

51. Capdevila X, Macaire P, Aknin P, et al. Patient-controlled perineural analgesia after ambulatory orthopedic surgery: a comparison of electronic versus elastomeric pumps. *Anesth Analg* 2003;**96**:414–7, table.

52. Utvoll J, Raeder J. *Anesth Analg* 2010;**110**; Feb 8: Epub.

53. Kerr DR, Kohan L. Local infiltration analgesia: a technique for the control of acute postoperative pain following knee and hip surgery: a case study of 325 patients. *Acta Orthop* 2008;**79**:174–83.

54. Ozgun H, Kurt MN, Kurt I, Cevikel MH. Comparison of local, spinal, and general anaesthesia for inguinal herniorrhaphy. *Eur J Surg* 2002;**168**:455–9.

55. Kehlet H, Dahl JB. Spinal anaesthesia for inguinal hernia repair? *Acta Anaesthesiol Scand* 2003;**47**:1–2.

56. Perk H, Soyupek S, Serel TA, et al. Tension-free vaginal tape for surgical treatment of stress urinary incontinence: two years follow-up. *Int J Urol* 2003;**10**:132–5.

57. van Berlo CL, Hess DA, Nijhuis PA, et al. Ambulatory sentinel node biopsy under local anaesthesia for patients with early breast cancer. *Eur J Surg Oncol* 2003;**29**:383–5.

58. Dahl V, Gierloff C, Omland E, Raeder JC. Spinal, epidural or propofol anaesthesia for out-patient knee arthroscopy? *Acta Anaesthesiol Scand* 1997;**41**:1341–5.

59. Mulroy MF, Salinas FV, Larkin KL, Polissar NL. Ambulatory surgery patients may be discharged before voiding after short-acting spinal and epidural anesthesia. *Anesthesiology* 2002;**97**:315–19.

60. Labas P, Ohradka B, Cambal M, et al. Haemorrhoidectomy in outpatient practice. *Eur J Surg* 2002;**168**:619–20.

61. Weinbroum AA, Lalayev G, Yashar T, et al. Combined pre-incisional oral dextromethorphan and epidural lidocaine for postoperative pain reduction and morphine sparing: a randomised double-blind study on day-surgery patients. *Anaesthesia* 2001;**56**:616–22.

62. Horlocker TT, Bajwa ZH, Ashraf Z, et al. Risk assessment of hemorrhagic complications associated with nonsteroidal antiinflammatory medications in ambulatory pain clinic patients undergoing epidural steroid injection. *Anesth Analg* 2002;**95**:1691–7, table.

63. Gilbert A, Owens BD, Mulroy MF. Epidural hematoma after outpatient epidural anesthesia. *Anesth Analg* 2002;**94**:77–8, table.

64. Buckenmaier CC, III, Steele SM, Nielsen KC, et al. Bilateral continuous paravertebral catheters for reduction mammoplasty. *Acta Anaesthesiol Scand* 2002;**46**:1042–5.

65. Weltz CR, Klein SM, Arbo JE, Greengrass RA. Paravertebral block anesthesia for inguinal hernia repair. *World J Surg* 2003;**27**:425–9.

66. Klein SM, Pietrobon R, Nielsen KC, et al. Paravertebral somatic nerve block compared with peripheral nerve blocks for outpatient inguinal herniorrhaphy. *Reg Anesth Pain Med* 2002;**27**:476–80.

67. Exadaktylos AK, Buggy DJ, Moriarty DC, et al. Can anesthetic technique for primary breast cancer surgery affect recurrence or metastasis? *Anesthesiology* 2006;**105**:660–4.

68. Moller JF, Nikolajsen L, Rodt SA, et al. Thoracic paravertebral block for breast cancer surgery: a randomized double-blind study. *Anesth Analg* 2007;**105**:1848–51, table.

69. Salinas FV, Liu SS. Spinal anaesthesia: local anaesthetics and adjuncts in the ambulatory setting. *Best Pract Res Clin Anaesthesiol* 2002;**16**:195–210.

70. Tong D, Wong J, Chung F, et al. Prospective study on incidence and functional impact of transient neurologic symptoms associated with 1% versus 5% hyperbaric lidocaine in short urologic procedures. *Anesthesiology* 2003;**98**:485–94.

71. Buckenmaier CC, III, Nielsen KC, Pietrobon R, et al. Small-dose intrathecal lidocaine versus ropivacaine for anorectal surgery in an ambulatory setting. *Anesth Analg* 2002;**95**:1253–7, table.

72. Lennox PH, Vaghadia H, Henderson C, et al. Small-dose selective spinal anesthesia for short-duration outpatient laparoscopy: recovery characteristics compared with desflurane anesthesia. *Anesth Analg* 2002;**94**:346–50, table.

73. Lopez-Soriano F, Lajarin B, Rivas F, et al. [Hyperbaric subarachnoid ropivacaine in ambulatory surgery: comparative study with hyperbaric bupivacaine.] *Rev Esp Anestesiol Reanim* 2002;**49**:71–5.

74. Whiteside JB, Burke D, Wildsmith JA. Comparison of ropivacaine 0.5% (in glucose 5%) with bupivacaine 0.5% (in glucose 8%) for spinal anaesthesia for elective surgery. *Br J Anaesth* 2003;**90**:304–8.

75. Breebaart MB, Vercauteren MP, Hoffmann VL, Adriaensen HA. Urinary bladder scanning after day-case arthroscopy under spinal anaesthesia: comparison between lidocaine, ropivacaine, and levobupivacaine. *Br J Anaesth* 2003;**90**:309–13.

76. Imarengiaye CO, Song D, Prabhu AJ, Chung F. Spinal anesthesia: functional balance is

impaired after clinical recovery. *Anesthesiology* 2003;**98**:511–15.

77. Gupta A, Axelsson K, Thorn SE, et al. Low-dose bupivacaine plus fentanyl for spinal anesthesia during ambulatory inguinal herniorrhaphy: a comparison between 6 mg and 7. 5 mg of bupivacaine. *Acta Anaesthesiol Scand* 2003;**47**:13–19.

78. Korhonen AM, Valanne JV, Jokela RM, et al. Intrathecal hyperbaric bupivacaine 3 mg + fentanyl 10 μg for outpatient knee arthroscopy with tourniquet. *Acta Anaesthesiol Scand* 2003;**47**:342–6.

79. De KM, Gautier P, Fanard L, et al. Intrathecal ropivacaine and clonidine for ambulatory knee arthroscopy: a dose-response study. *Anesthesiology* 2001;**94**:574–8.

80. Merivirta R, Kuusniemi K, Jaakkola P, et al. Unilateral spinal anaesthesia for outpatient surgery: a comparison between hyperbaric bupivacaine and bupivacaine-clonidine combination. *Acta Anaesthesiol Scand* 2009;**53**:788–93.

81. Hendriks MP, de Weert CJ, Snoeck MM, et al. Plain articaine or prilocaine for spinal anaesthesia in day-case knee arthroscopy: a double-blind randomized trial. *Br J Anaesth* 2009;**102**:259–63.

82. Sell A, Tein T, Pitkanen M. Spinal 2-chloroprocaine: effective dose for ambulatory surgery. *Acta Anaesthesiol Scand* 2008;**52**:695–9.

83. Williams BA, Kentor ML, Vogt MT, et al. Femoral-sciatic nerve blocks for complex outpatient knee surgery are associated with less postoperative pain before same-day discharge: a review of 1,200 consecutive cases from the period 1996–1999. *Anesthesiology* 2003;**98**:1206–13.

84. Provenzano DA, Viscusi ER, Adams SB, Jr., et al. Safety and efficacy of the popliteal fossa nerve block when utilized for foot and ankle surgery. *Foot Ankle Int* 2002;**23**:394–9.

85. Pandin P, Vandesteene A, D'Hollander A. Sciatic nerve blockade in the supine position: a novel approach. *Can J Anaesth* 2003;**50**:52–6.

86. Casati A, Borghi B, Fanelli G, et al. A double-blinded, randomized comparison of either 0.5% levobupivacaine or 0.5% ropivacaine for sciatic nerve block. *Anesth Analg* 2002;**94**:987–90, table.

87. Singelyn FJ. Single-injection applications for foot and ankle surgery. *Best Pract Res Clin Anaesthesiol* 2002;**16**:247–54.

88. Clough TM, Sandher D, Bale RS, Laurence AS. The use of a local anesthetic foot block in patients undergoing outpatient bony forefoot surgery: a prospective randomized controlled trial. *J Foot Ankle Surg* 2003;**42**:24–9.

89. Sia S, Lepri A, Campolo MC, Fiaschi R. Four-injection brachial plexus block using peripheral nerve stimulator: a comparison between axillary and humeral approaches. *Anesth Analg* 2002;**95**:1075–9, table.

90. Deleuze A, Gentili ME, Marret E, et al. A comparison of a single-stimulation lateral infraclavicular plexus block with a triple-stimulation axillary block. *Reg Anesth Pain Med* 2003;**28**:89–94.

91. Candido KD, Winnie AP, Ghaleb AH, et al. Buprenorphine added to the local anesthetic for axillary brachial plexus block prolongs postoperative analgesia. *Reg Anesth Pain Med* 2002;**27**:162–7.

92. Krenn H, Deusch E, Balogh B, et al. Increasing the injection volume by dilution improves the onset of motor blockade, but not sensory blockade of ropivacaine for brachial plexus block. *Eur J Anaesthesiol* 2003;**20**:21–5.

93. Sandhu NS, Capan LM. Ultrasound-guided infraclavicular brachial plexus block. *Br J Anaesth* 2002;**89**:254–9.

94. Tran de QH, Russo G, Munoz L, et al. A prospective, randomized comparison between ultrasound-guided supraclavicular, infraclavicular, and axillary brachial plexus blocks. *Reg Anesth Pain Med* 2009;**34**:366–71.

95. Tran de QH, Munoz L, Russo G, Finlayson RJ. Ultrasonography and stimulating perineural catheters for nerve blocks: a review of the evidence. *Can J Anaesth* 2008;**55**:447–57.

96. Aasbo V, Thuen A, Raeder J. Improved long-lasting postoperative analgesia, recovery function and patient satisfaction after

inguinal hernia repair with inguinal field block compared with general anesthesia. *Acta Anaesthesiol Scand* 2002;**46**:674–8.

97. Ghani KR, McMillan R, Paterson-Brown S. Transient femoral nerve palsy following ilio-inguinal nerve blockade for day case inguinal hernia repair. *J R Coll Surg Edinb* 2002;**47**:626–9.

98. Klein SM, Nielsen KC, Greengrass RA, et al. Ambulatory discharge after long-acting peripheral nerve blockade: 2382 blocks with ropivacaine. *Anesth Analg* 2002;**94**:65–70, table.

99. Herr GP, Conner JT, Katz RL, et al. Diazepam and droperidol as i.v. premedicants. *Br J Anaesth* 1979;**51**:537–42.

100. Servin FS, Raeder JC, Merle JC, et al. Remifentanil sedation compared with propofol during regional anaesthesia. *Acta Anaesthesiol Scand* 2002;**46**:309–15.

101. Servin F. Ambulatory anesthesia for the obese patient. *Curr Opin Anaesthesiol* 2006;**19**:597–9.

102. Smith I, Avramov MN, White PF. A comparison of propofol and remifentanil during monitored anesthesia care. *J Clin Anesth* 1997;**9**:148–54.

103. Riviere PJ. Peripheral kappa-opioid agonists for visceral pain. *Br J Pharmacol* 2004;**141**:1331–4.

104. Bennett J, Wren KR, Haas R. Opioid use during the perianesthesia period: nursing implications. *J Perianesth Nurs* 2001;**16**:255–8.

105. Lallo A, Billard V, Bourgain JL. A comparison of propofol and remifentanil target-controlled infusions to facilitate fiberoptic nasotracheal intubation. *Anesth Analg* 2009;**108**:852–7.

106. Akcaboy ZN, Akcaboy EY, Albayrak D, et al. Can remifentanil be a better choice than propofol for colonoscopy during monitored anesthesia care? *Acta Anaesthesiol Scand* 2006;**50**:736–41.

107. Skipsey IG, Colvin JR, Mackenzie N, Kenny GN. Sedation with propofol during surgery under local blockade. Assessment of a target-controlled infusion system. *Anaesthesia* 1993;**48**:210–13.

108. Church JA, Stanton PD, Kenny GN, Anderson JR. Propofol for sedation during endoscopy: assessment of a computer-controlled infusion system. *Gastrointest Endosc* 1991;**37**:175–9.

109. Nieuwenhuijs DJ, Olofsen E, Romberg RR, et al. Response surface modeling of remifentanil-propofol interaction on cardiorespiratory control and bispectral index. *Anesthesiology* 2003;**98**:312–22.

110. Gerlach AT, Dasta JF. Dexmedetomidine: an updated review. *Ann Pharmacother* 2007;**41**:245–52.

111. Ekman A, Lindholm ML, Lennmarken C, Sandin R. Reduction in the incidence of awareness using BIS monitoring. *Acta Anaesthesiol Scand* 2004;**48**:20–6.

112. Gan TJ, Glass PS, Windsor A, Payne F, Rosow C, Sebel P, Manberg P. Bispectral index monitoring allows faster emergence and improved recovery from propofol, alfentanil, and nitrous oxide anesthesia. BIS Utility Study Group. *Anesthesiology* 1997;**87**:808–15.

113. Kuratani N, Oi Y. Greater incidence of emergence agitation in children after sevoflurane anesthesia as compared with halothane: a meta-analysis of randomized controlled trials. *Anesthesiology* 2008;**109**:225–32.

114. Mayer J, Boldt J, Rohm KD, et al. Desflurane anesthesia after sevoflurane inhaled induction reduces severity of emergence agitation in children undergoing minor ear-nose-throat surgery compared with sevoflurane induction and maintenance. *Anesth Analg* 2006;**102**:400–4.

115. Einarsson SG, Cerne A, Bengtsson A, et al. Respiration during emergence from anaesthesia with desflurane/N$_2$O vs. desflurane/air for gynaecological laparoscopy. *Acta Anaesthesiol Scand* 1998;**42**:1192–8.

116. Raeder J. Bariatric procedures as day/short stay surgery: is it possible and reasonable? *Curr Opin Anaesthesiol* 2007;**20**:508–12.

117. Servin F. Ambulatory anesthesia for the obese patient. *Curr Opin Anaesthesiol* 2006;**19**:597–9.

118. Talab HF, Zabani IA, Abdelrahman HS, et al. Intraoperative ventilatory strategies for prevention of pulmonary atelectasis in obese patients undergoing laparoscopic bariatric surgery. *Anesth Analg* 2009;**109**:1511–16.

119. De Baerdemaeker LE, Struys MM, Jacobs S, et al. Optimization of desflurane administration in morbidly obese patients: a comparison with sevoflurane using an 'inhalation bolus' technique. *Br J Anaesth* 2003;**91**:638–50.

120. Ahonen J. Day surgery and thromboembolic complications: time for structured assessment and prophylaxis. *Curr Opin Anaesthesiol* 2007;**20**:535–9.

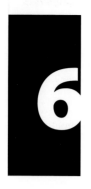

6 Postoperative care

Postoperative pain
Pain physiology

Pain is a subjective and unpleasant experience resulting from tissue damage or potential (threatening) tissue damage and is mediated through pain receptors and pain nerve fibers, also called nociceptive stimulation. Surgery may provoke pain by three important mechanisms (Figure 6.1):

1. Stimulation of peripheral nerve fibers and receptors in the surgical field, either by direct mechanical stimulation or through a change in the chemical environment: hypoxia, acidity, heat, cold, or release of potent proteins from damaged cells and inflammation.

2. Cutting of small nerve fibers and destruction of neurons. As nerve fibers are ubiquitous in the body, even slight surgical trauma will result in some nerve fiber damage. This means that surgical trauma itself has a neuropathic pain component, as a traumatized nerve fiber means a traumatized neuron, and damaged neurons may generate pain themselves or respond to stimulation abnormally.

3. Surgery always damages normal cells of many types. Potent proteins and enzymes are then activated and liberated from these damaged cells. They cause inflammation at the injury site and also have systemic effects in the spinal cord and brain once distributed by the circulation. For instance, it has been shown that cyclooxygenase (COX) is activated to produce prostaglandins, inflammation, and pain in the wound area and also the spinal cord and brain following distribution of proteins via the circulation.

Efficient loco-regional anesthesia will attenuate the localized wound inflammation, block nerve transmission, and (temporarily) stop the pain mediated by damaged neurons; despite this, the proteins released systemically will remain active.

With general anesthesia the patient is protected from feeling pain during the procedure, but the pain-stimulating mechanisms will still start at the same time as surgery. Tissue trauma will initiate localized inflammation and enforced pain stimulation (primary hyperalgesia). Continuous and strong pain stimulation at the spinal dorsal horn mobilizes N-methyl-D-aspartate (NMDA) receptors and COX enzymes, among others, to induce a secondary hyperalgesia. Thus it has been postulated, and heavily debated, whether appropriate anti-nociceptive (e.g., analgesic) treatment started before the occurrence of trauma, so-called pre-emptive analgesia, will result in less pain later on, simply because the pain-generating mechanisms are attenuated. The concept of the pre-emptive effect means that giving an analgesic preoperatively will be more efficient than giving the same drug and dose at the end of anesthesia before emergence. While demonstrated convincingly in animals, the results

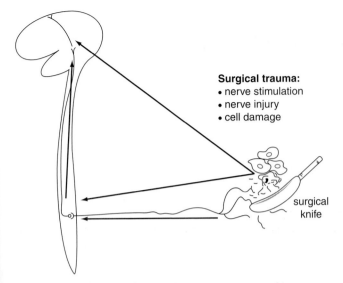

Surgical trauma:
- nerve stimulation
- nerve injury
- cell damage

surgical knife

Figure 6.1. Modes of surgical trauma and pain. The knife is touching and cutting nerve fibers, and destroying cells. The nerve fibers signal to a synapse in the spinal dorsal horn, which is relayed further to synapse first in the thalamus and subsequently to cortical structures; subjective pain is felt if the patient is awake. Cell destruction results in peripheral inflammation and systemic distribution of pain initiators and mediators to the spine and brain.

in humans are much more inconclusive. Nevertheless, the meta-analysis by Ong et al. [1] concluded that there was a true pre-emptive effect with epidural analgesia, local anesthesia, and nonsteroidal anti-inflammatory drugs (NSAIDS), whereas the association was uncertain with NMDA inhibitors and not present with opioids. An important issue in this discussion may be that, in order to work, the pre-emptive attenuation of nociceptive stimulation should not only be given prior to surgery, but should also be maintained throughout the whole procedure and also for some time postoperatively. It has been shown that strong nociceptive stimulation will continue for many hours and days after the end of surgery from the wound area, even if kept rested. Movement may be viewed as new, small trauma in unhealed tissue [2].

The best way to treat acute pain is to minimize tissue injury and to prevent or reduce inflammatory and neuropathic stimulation. Administration of nonopioid analgesics can reduce inflammatory responses and peripheral neuropathic sensitization, thereby minimizing nociceptive pain and also opioid dose requirements. Prophylactic, preventative measures designed to minimize tissue injury (noninvasive surgery) and inflammation (NSAIDs and other anti-inflammatory agents) are important in this context. Gentle and minimally traumatic surgery should be the aim, e.g., endoscopic procedures are associated with significantly less tissue injury and are generally less painful than open invasive surgery. Also, nonpharmacologic measures to further reduce tissue damage, inflammation, and nerve stimulation may be provided, particularly when the pain-provoking process is ongoing as in the early postoperative period. Examples are limb elevation, compression, and localized cooling to reduce inflammation and edema.

Analgesics have variable sites of activity and can interact with receptors, as well as local and humoral mediators in injured tissues (Figure 6.2), or on nerves and nerve endings that transmit nociceptive stimuli to the central nervous system. They also act on pain-transmitting mechanisms in the spinal dorsal horn (Figure 6.3) and at cortical sites that process subjective discomfort.

Peripheral nociception

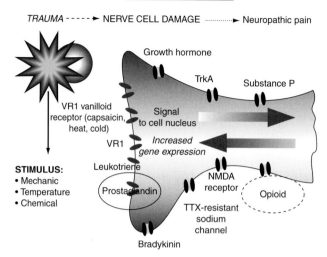

Figure 6.2. Schematic view of a peripheral nerve ending. Many receptors are activated by proteins and molecules. Prostaglandin synthesis may be reduced by NSAIDs and steroids, with subsequent less receptor binding and less excitation. The opioid receptors are only expressed in tissues in the presence of inflammation, and, if present, the stimulation of these by endogenous opioids or opioid drugs may contribute to the reduced excitability of the nerve.

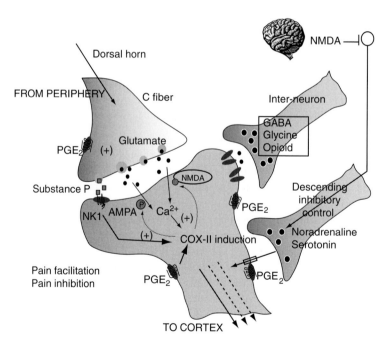

Figure 6.3. Important pain transmission mechanisms in the spinal dorsal horn. An impulse from the periphery will liberate glutamate, which will activate the α-amino-3-hydroxyl-5-methyl-4-isoxazole-propionate (AMPA) receptor postsynaptically and transmit the impulse further to the thalamus and cortex. If the peripheral impulse is strong enough and long-lasting (repetitive) the NMDA channels may also open and activate Ca^{2+} influx, which will reinforce the postsynaptic signal. Also the COX-II enzyme may be activated and contribute to reinforced transmission. The transmission may be inhibited by opioid and also γ-aminobutyric acid (GABA), as well as by descending inhibitory pathways with serotonin and noradrenaline release. NMDA receptor stimulation in the brain may inhibit the descending inhibition, thus an NMDA antagonist will reinforce the descending inhibition as well as act to block the activated NMDA receptor in the dorsal horn.

The role of opioids

The opioids are among the oldest of pain relievers known to humans, and they remain the cornerstone of acute pain management in patients with moderately severe to severe symptoms. Their benefits include a rapid onset of action, no upper limit of efficacy, many modes of administration, and low cost. Well-known side-effects such as nausea, vomiting, pruritus, constipation, and respiratory depression limit their use and may impose significant morbidity. Most opioids have a high degree of first-pass metabolism in the liver making oral dosing unpredictable. Opioid-induced sedation, i.e., hypnosis and anxiolysis, may be of benefit in some situations; but these effects are unreliable and some patients may experience excessive obtundation, sleep apnea, airway obstruction, confusion, and impaired cognition. Whereas opioids may be titrated to effectively relieve pain at rest, they are not so efficient in controlling incident pain during mobilization. This limitation may be problematic in settings where patients require physiotherapy or physical activity during rehabilitation and recovery. Further, the opioids may disturb the natural pattern of sleep, with reduced fraction of REM sleep after dosing and catch-up and restless nights later on. Recently, focus has also been on the immunosuppressive action of long-term opioid use, potentially harmful in terms of increased risk of infection and tumor spread [3].

Although tolerance and dependency are well recognized problems with continued opioid use, the development of hyperalgesia or reduced threshold for discomfort from pain stimuli has also become recognized as a clinical concern. Such hyperalgesia has been reported after just a few hours of exposure. Opioids do not seem to be effective for pre-emptive analgesia and do not seem to protect against development of chronic pain in the same way as some other analgesics may possibly do [1].

Thus, the role of opioid postoperatively after ambulatory surgery will be as a rescue drug when needed on top of an otherwise multimodal nonopioid regimen.

Principles of employing nonopioid analgesics

A major problem with many of the nonopioid modalities is the ceiling of effect or lack of strong analgesic effect. Thus, it is an important concept to combine them optimally, so-called *multimodal analgesia*. The idea is that even a weak analgesic (such as paracetamol) may contribute to the overall analgesic effect. Given together with other weak or medium strength analgesics they may together be fairly strong. The multimodal concept is also supported by the idea of using drugs with different targets along the nociceptive pathway: from peripheral trauma, through nerves, to spinal cord, to the thalamus and brain. The target may be to attenuate or block a synaptic stimulation or ion channel opening, to block conduction in nerves, but may also be to enhance the body's own mechanisms of controlling and reducing pain such as with the opioids and α2 agonists. A further issue with multimodality is to keep the side-effects down because each drug may have different and mild side-effects, which are not additive when the drugs are combined, in contrast to the analgesic effect, which is.

Timing is another issue: pre-emptive use is controversial (see above), whereas there is certainly good reason to give these drugs before the patient feels pain and to then continue with a prophylactic approach for as long as is needed. This is both because it is better for the patient not to have to wait for the analgesics until they first experience pain, and also because pain experienced without any analgesics on board may grow strong and difficult to treat.

Nonopioid analgesic drugs

Local anesthesia

Local anesthesia is an efficient nonopioid pharmacological approach to postoperative analgesia. Local anesthesia is used for both neural blockade and infiltration.

The use of neuronal blockade for surgery is effective for postoperative pain and has an opioid-sparing effect [4]. Different infiltration techniques have been shown to be pain-reducing and opioid-sparing after cholecystectomy [5], inguinal hernia repair [6], breast surgery [7], gynecologic laparotomies [8], and orthopedic [9] and anorectal [10] surgery. A study has shown a beneficial effect from infiltration of local anesthesia in the trocar entrance areas after laparoscopic procedures [11]. Instillation of local anesthesia without infiltrating has also been proven to be efficacious. Topical analgesia with lidocaine aerosol was found to be highly effective after inguinal herniorrhaphy [12], and instillation of bupivacaine with epinephrine or lidocaine during laparoscopy reduces postoperative scapular pain [13]. Topical administration of local anesthesia has excellent analgesic properties after ambulatory circumcision in children [14]. In addition to the traditional effects of local anesthesia, the amide local anesthetics seem to have a long-lasting anti-inflammatory effect, thereby blocking the postoperative inflammatory process at the surgical site [15,16]. Although the benefits are evident, more studies are needed to evaluate optimal methods for infiltration and topical administration [17]. There is also a lack of clinical studies investigating different techniques of wound infiltration with combinations of other pharmacological agents and analgesic methods [18]. Difficulties in infiltrating all relevant structures, especially after major surgery, limit the efficacy of wound infiltration. The short duration of the different local anesthetic agents is also limiting. An ideal local anesthetic drug in the postoperative setting would be one providing ultra-long analgesia. There are promising results from animal studies showing that the duration of an anesthetic block can be considerably prolonged by increasing the viscosity of the local anesthetic [19]. Encapsulation in liposomes prolongs the duration of the local anesthetics in animal models [20]. Another interesting field of research is the inclusion of local anesthesia in monoolein water systems. This technique uses the monoolein water system to give a product which is liquid at room temperature and highly viscous at body temperature, thus providing an easily injectable slow-release system [21].

Paracetamol

Paracetamol is a well-established analgesic drug for the postoperative period, and is widely used as a basis for postoperative pain treatment. The need for opioid analgesia has typically been reduced by 20–30% when combined with a regular regimen of oral or rectal paracetamol. The exact mechanism of action is still debated; it seems to have some indirect effect on the cyclooxygenase system, but also a central component. Paracetamol easily crosses the blood–brain barrier and has also been shown to interact with the type-3 5-hydroxytryptamine- (5HT3-) blocking drugs [22–24]. Paracetamol, given as a single dose of 1000 mg, has a number-needed-to-treat (NNT) of 3.6, which in one study was better than for instance tramadol 100 mg or the combination of acetylsalicylic acid 650 mg and codeine 60 mg [25]. In comparison with clinical doses of NSAIDs it probably has less analgesic potency, but seems to have an additional analgesic effect when given in combination [26,27]. For instance, the combination of diclofenac and paracetamol for postoperative pain after oral surgery enhances and prolongs the analgesic effect compared with either of the two drugs used alone [28]. Studies on children indicate that paracetamol has good analgesic properties when serum levels of 10–20 mg/l are achieved, and this level can be reached with a dosage of 40 mg/kg orally [29]. The use of rectal administration for children is widely used, but the recommended dosages are often insufficient. Studies have shown a dose/response analgesic efficacy in the postoperative pediatric patient up to a single dose of 60 mg/kg without any side-effects [30]. Bremerich et al. have measured the mean paracetamol concentration after rectal administration to 3.5 mg/l after 20 mg/kg and 6.2 mg/l after 40 mg/kg, with poor analgesic effect in the postoperative period [31]. When compared with oral paracetamol, rectal administration has a slower onset with a maximum serum concentration at 2–2.5 h as compared to 0.6 h for tablets, and also a lower peak serum level [32]. This should be taken into consideration when suppositories are used for postoperative pain treatment. Clearly, a single rectal dose of 40–60 mg/kg paracetamol seems safe in children. If paracetamol is used rectally in adults, the first dosage should probably exceed the per oral dosage by 50%. An intravenous precursor of paracetamol, propacetamol, has also been in use for some years. One gram of the precursor readily converts into 0.5 g paracetamol. Propacetamol has proven to be efficacious as postoperative analgesia. After orthopedic surgery it has been demonstrated that propacetamol reduces the postoperative opioid requirement by 46% [33].

As propacetamol may ache in the veins [34] and an intravenous paracetamol parent drug has come available, this will replace propacetamol for iv use [35]. As paracetamol is almost 100% absorbed by the oral route, there are indications not to reduce the dose by iv use. A study of paracetamol 1 g versus 2 g iv in adults showed a better analgesic effect of the 2 g dose [36].

There are concerns regarding the side-effects of paracetamol, such as a potential genotoxic effect [37] and renal toxicity, when used in combination with NSAIDs in vulnerable patients [38]. Also, the therapeutic window of paracetamol is low, and even small amounts of paracetamol overdosage can result in liver damage [39]. When used in analgesic doses, however, there is no evidence of genotoxicity [40]. Paracetamol in combination with NSAIDs should, however, be used with caution in patients requiring a high level of prostaglandins to maintain adequate renal perfusion, such as hypovolemic patients and elderly patients with renal failure. When used alone, paracetamol is considered safe even in this group of patients.

There have been some reports of a diminished effect of paracetamol when ondansetron is given first [41]. This probably has to do with a pharmacodynamic interaction at the 5HT3 receptor. The clinical importance of this in patients has not yet been studied much, and it is also unclear whether the interaction will be present if paracetamol is given before the 5HT3 antagonist.

In summary, paracetamol is efficacious as a basic postoperative analgesic. Used in combination with a NSAID, paracetamol seems to give additional analgesia. The use of iv paracetamol enables a more flexible use of this drug in the perioperative setting.

Nonsteroidal anti-inflammatory drugs (NSAIDs)

The arachidonic acid cascade system is the most important phospholipid-derived messenger system and plays a key regulatory role in cell physiology. Oxidation of arachidonic acid via the cyclooxygenase (COX) pathway generates a series of prostaglandins and thromboxanes, many of which play a substantial role in the perception of pain. Prostaglandins and thromboxanes are generated by tissue trauma and mediate nociception by sensitization of peripheral nociceptors in synergy with other chemical mediators. NSAIDs block the synthesis of prostaglandins by inhibition of the enzyme COX [42] (Figure 6.4). However, NSAIDs also have prostaglandin-independent effects in the periphery [43,44], and research

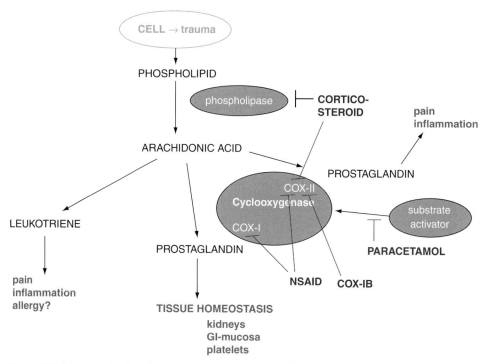

Figure 6.4. Schematic drawing of prostaglandin's role in pain and physiology.
Cell trauma releases phospholipid, which is degraded by phospholipase to arachidonic acid, which will subsequently be degraded by cyclooxygenase to prostaglandin. COX-I activity normally produces prostaglandin, which keeps kidney vessels open by hypovolemia, aids platelet activity in clotting when activated during bleeding, and has a role in the production of mucus to protect the gut and intestinal mucosal surfaces. COX-II is more strongly activated by trauma and cell damage, and is responsible for pain and inflammation. Corticosteroids inhibit both phospholipase and COX-II. Traditional NSAIDs inhibit both COX-I and COX-II, whereas the COX-II inhibitors inhibit just COX-II. Paracetamol has (among other effects) an indirect effect on COX synthesis as well.

suggests that a substantial part of the analgesia provided by this group of drugs is centrally mediated [45]. NSAIDs are well-known analgesics with opioid-sparing effects [46]. They are highly efficacious in the treatment of postoperative pain after orthopedic and major gynecologic surgery [47]. For certain types of pain with reduced opioid sensitivity, such as pain from bone metastases, gall bladder and urinary spasm pain, NSAIDs are particularly beneficial [48]. The injectable forms of NSAIDs, such as ketorolac, ketoprofen, and diclofenac, enable perioperative analgesia without the many side-effects of opioids. In children, NSAIDs have been successfully used for postoperative analgesia and other painful conditions such as acute otitis media [49–51].

However, the use of NSAIDs is limited by contraindications and potentially severe side-effects. Prostaglandin E_2 and prostacyclin (PGI_2) are essential for the production of the gastric-mucosa-protecting mucus, and gastrointestinal bleeding is a well known complication of NSAIDs [52]. Renal impairment is another risk, especially in patients who are dependent on a high level of renal prostaglandins, such as elderly patients with arteriosclerosis and hypovolemic patients. In cohort studies, however, short-term use of NSAIDs (i.e., less than 5 days) in patients under 75 years of age did not increase the incidence of renal failure or gastrointestinal bleeding [53,54]. Acute bronchospasm is also a potential side-effect of NSAIDs, and 8–20% of patients with asthma will experience bronchospasm after using NSAIDs [55]. A major controversial issue is the combination of NSAIDs with low-molecular-weight heparins for venous thrombosis prophylaxis. Although NSAIDs' antiplatelet effect is unlikely to produce perioperative bleeding complications by itself [56], there are some concerns about the combination [57].

The cyclooxygenase enzyme exists as at least two different isoenzymes: COX-I and COX-II [58]. The COX-I isoenzyme is the constitutive form with physiologic functions in normal homeostasis, while COX-II is the inducible form. During inflammation COX-II is induced and upregulated, thereby producing high levels of prostanoids, whereas the COX-I levels remain almost unaffected. However, the lungs, kidneys, and neural tissue have a high level of COX-II even in the absence of external stimuli. NSAIDs with a high COX-II specificity theoretically have a beneficial effect on inflammation and pain perception without affecting the homeostatic functions of prostaglandins. Drugs with higher potency against COX-II than COX-I will produce fewer side-effects. The potency of NSAIDs against either enzyme can be expressed as shown in Figure 6.5. A drug with a high COX-I affinity, such as piroxicam, induces more gastrointestinal side-effects than celecoxib, which has a high COX-II affinity [59]. It is generally agreed that the clinical analgesic effects of NSAIDs and COX-II inhibitors are similar, but there are experimental and also clinical data supporting the view that incisional pain is strongly mediated by COX-I activation in the spinal cord [60].

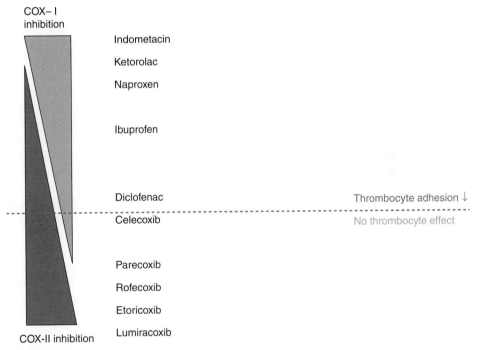

Figure 6.5. The relative inhibitory effects on COX-I and COX-II of different NSAIDs. Ketorolac and naproxen are almost pure COX-I inhibitors, whereas parecoxib and etoricoxib are almost pure COX-II inhibitors. Although diclofenac and celecoxib are not very different, diclofenac reduces the adhesive-aggregating effect of thrombocytes, whereas celecoxib has no such efficacy in clinical doses.

In a study comparing etoricoxib with ketorolac we also found that ketorolac had a stronger initial analgesic effect than etoricoxib [61]. Clinically, the impression is that iv ketorolac may have a clear additional effect on patients already on a maximally effective dose of COX-II inhibitor. There is also some speculation that ketorolac has effects other than COX inhibition for analgesia.

While traditional NSAIDs remain the cornerstone for postoperative analgesia, the new COX-II selective drugs, (i.e., celecoxib, etoricoxib, and parecoxib), also called COX inhibitors, have some beneficial features. Apart from having fewer gastrointestinal side-effects, they do not influence bleeding tendency, and are safer in patients with allergy and asthma. Etoricoxib in particular has strong receptor binding such that dosing is only needed once per day, thus patient compliance is better and there is less breakthrough pain. However, they may still cause renal failure in the fragile or hypovolemic patient, they may cause slight hypertension and fluid retention with short-term use, and increase the risk of cardiovascular morbidity with regular use over many months.

The cardiovascular effects of the different COX inhibitors seem to vary greatly. Rofecoxib was worst in this regard (and has been withdrawn from the market), whereas a large 1- to 2-year study of diclofenac versus etoricoxib did not reveal any difference between the two in terms of cardiovascular morbidity [62]. The only study demonstrating coronary problems with short-term use of COX inhibitors is a 10-day study of parecoxib and valdecoxib in coronary bypass surgery patients [63]. These patients represent a specific model, because they have postoperative wound healing taking place inside freshly operated coronary arteries, and the results from this study cannot be extrapolated to noncardiac ambulatory surgery [64].

Whereas diclofenac and ibuprofen are probably quite similar to the COX inhibitors in terms of cardiovascular risk, they may differ from naproxen, which is a fairly pure COX-I inhibitor and has been demonstrated to have a minor antithrombotic effect and potentially fewer cardiovascular problems with long-term use.

Another issue with traditional NSAIDs is bleeding tendency. The thrombocyte adhesive function is reduced and increased bleeding and bruising may be seen, clinically demonstrated after gynecologic surgery, orthopedic surgery, and tonsillectomy [65,66]. It is also a concern of many plastic surgeons and others that bruising and hematoma formation occur more readily after NSAID use, although there are no prospective randomized studies supporting these statements. Although the bleeding issue is probably not a significant one in terms of major morbidity, it may be an argument for using the COX-II inhibitors as they have no such effect on platelets. An alternative strategy is to postpone traditional NSAIDs until there is good hemostasis, because the thrombocyte adhesion is more important in primary bleeding and clot formation than when hemostasis is established and stable.

A final controversy with all the NSAIDs, and also glucocorticoids, is their inhibitory action on all kinds of inflammatory cells, immunostimulation, and tissue healing. The basic concern has been raised by orthopedic surgeons because reduced bone healing has been demonstrated in animal models [67] and also in a clinical model of spinal fusion surgery with a high dose of ketorolac for 3–5 days [68]. Nevertheless, these analgesics may be particularly useful in the orthopedic setting where pain may be quite strong during the necessary and beneficial mobilization after surgery. The conclusion in different centers varies from allowing full use in all orthopedic patients for up to 5–7 days, to abandoning all use in patients with fractured bone or tendon sutures [67]. Our conclusion is to allow 1–3 days of use in ambulatory orthopedic surgery cases unless there is a special indication for not doing so (pseudarthrosis, healing problems expected, heavy smoking, high age, diabetes, etc.). If there is a good indication (i.e., strong pain and good effect) the treatment may be continued for up to 7 days, but then there should be a careful evaluation of the pros and cons before going on further. But again, this has to be discussed with the orthopedic surgeons as scientific and clinical evidence is lacking in this area.

In spite of the potentially dangerous side-effects of NSAIDs, they are of great value in the perioperative period and are usually well tolerated as long as the drug is used in appropriate doses and contraindications are respected.

Glucocorticoids

The glucocorticoids are naturally occurring hormones in the body, with a diurnal variation in circulating levels with mobilization and increased circulating levels during trauma and stress. Typically about 25–50 mg cortisone is secreted during a normal 24-h period [69]. The clinically analgesic effect of stress hormones has long been acknowledged [70,71]; for instance, during combat situations where the pain threshold seems to be significantly elevated, possibly partly due to glucocorticoids and other stress hormones. It has also been shown that animals with elevated levels of endogenous glucocorticoids experience less pain than others [72].

The therapeutic benefits associated with glucocorticoids have not been tested or documented as well as have other pain relievers partly due to the fact that glucocorticoids are inexpensive and old. Also, the fear of side-effects and the lack of exact knowledge of their analgesic mechanisms have limited the introduction of this class of drug into routine clinical use. However, this lack of interest may be challenged as ongoing research is performed on membrane-bound glucocorticoid receptors and more selective and potentially safer steroid agonists [73].

Effect mechanisms

Glucocorticoids act by binding to a class of nuclear receptors (corticosteroid receptors). Upon binding to the receptor transfer (chaperone) protein, the drug–receptor complex diffuses into the nucleus of the cell and binds to DNA, initiating the production of proteins and enzymes with subsequent clinical effects [74–76]. Traditional pharmacokinetic parameters are not appropriate for describing glucocorticoid pharmacodynamics, since DNA activation is associated with significant latency to effect. For this reason onset is typically delayed, with maximum glucocorticoid effects observed after 3–4 h or more [77, 78]. For the same reason, the duration of clinical effect is prolonged and does not correlate with plasma concentrations of the drug. In general, effects on cellular processes will continue for hours to days, despite the complete clearance of drug from plasma.

Some direct cellular membrane effects of glucocorticoids have also been suggested [73]. The rapid membrane stabilization from glucocorticoids during anaphylactic reactions, and a study by Romundstad et al. showing an analgesic effect within 1 h of administration are clinically supportive of these non-DNA-mediated effects of glucocorticoids [79].

Molecular actions of glucocorticoids

The family of steroid molecules includes potent hormones necessary for normal homeostasis and growth of the human body [71]. The glucocorticoids have virtually no sex hormonal effects, but some of them may still have slight mineralocorticoid properties resulting in renal sodium and water retention [80]. There are also some reports of increased blood sugar levels, especially in diabetic patients [81]. The major effects of the glucocorticoid subclass of steroid hormones are linked with the inflammatory response; including inhibition of inflammatory gene expression and stimulation of anti-inflammatory gene expression. Important mediators include COX-II inhibition [82], tumor necrosis factor (TNF) inhibition, and leukocyte inhibition, in both peripheral injured tissue and the spinal dorsal horn and central nervous system. As part of this general anti-inflammatory action, glucocorticoids also have direct effects on blood capillaries, with decreased permeability and reduced vasodilatation.

A general anti-inflammatory action may be very important for pain reduction per se, by reducing local tissue pressure and limiting the release of potent pain mediators. The glucocorticoids have also been shown to have direct effects on pain neurons and receptors. They reduce neuropeptide release, inhibit signal transmission in C-fibers, and stimulate the secretion of endogenous endorphins.

Clinical actions of glucocorticoids

The well-known clinical effects of glucocorticoids include anti-inflammation, anti-edema, anti-allergic, and antipyretic effects. Also analgesia and anti-emetic effects [83] are well documented although the mechanisms, especially of anti-emesis, are less well understood. The glucocorticoids frequently induce a slight feeling of euphoria and alertness, being documented in the postoperative setting as less sleepiness when these drugs are used [84]. The patient may sometimes describe a sensation of more "energy" when these drugs are used and also increased appetite may be beneficial in this setting. In contrast, there also are reports on restlessness, dysphoria, and even rare cases of abrupt psychosis [85], when glucocorticoids are used in the postoperative setting. Less postoperative shivering has been observed and fewer cardiac arrhythmias, although the latter effect is only shown in some studies whereas others have been negative [84].

With prolonged use of these drugs there is a long list of nonbeneficial effects, resulting from a generalized reduction in tissue growth, deprived cellular activation, as well as decreased bone healing and wound healing. The clinical manifestations may be: wound rupture, non-fusion of fractures, gastric ulceration and perforation, skin vulnerability and wound formation, and poor infection control. Also hormonal side-effects may develop, such as moon-face appearance, sexual hormone dysfunction, mental disturbances, and hyperglycemia.

Clinical analgesic action

The postoperative analgesic effect of glucocorticoids has been well documented [70,71,77,79,86–92]. Compared with other analgesics, the onset of clinical effect is generally delayed. In our experience, a minor analgesic effect is evident during the first 2–3 h following administration of 16 mg dexamethasone to patients recovering from breast surgery. This correlates with previous reports of delayed onset of effect. Aasboe et al. were not able to demonstrate any analgesic effect from 12 mg betamethasone until 3 h postoperatively [77]. In a laparoscopic surgical trial, Coloma et al. found that the anti-emetic effect of dexamethasone was more pronounced after discharge than in the immediate 3 h postoperatively [78]. Alternatively, Romundstad et al. reported that the onset of postsurgical analgesia provided by 125 mg iv methylprednisolone was evident at 60 min after administration [89]. This is in accordance with experimental and clinical evidence suggesting that glucocorticoids may have rapid and direct nongenomic actions on cellular membranes [76]. The duration of analgesic effect provided by single doses of iv glucocorticoids may be prolonged. In the study of Hval and coworkers 16 mg dexamethasone provided analgesia for 3 days after breast surgery [93].

Also Romundstad and coworkers [79] found that a single dose of 125 mg methylpredniso-lone provided measurable analgesic effects for 3 days. Similarly, Bisgaard et al. reported that a single dose of dexamethasone 8 mg significantly reduced pain intensity up to 1 week follow-ing laparoscopic surgery [88]. The plasma elimination half-life of dexamethasone is only about 6 h [94], thus there seem to be ongoing drug effects for a significant period after drug clearance from the plasma.

The optimal dose for glucocorticoid analgesic effect is not established, as controlled dose-finding studies have not been performed. For the anti-emetic effect of glucocorticoids, two dose-finding studies of dexamethasone have given conflicting results: in the study of Liu et al. [95] 2.5 mg was effective, whereas Lee et al. found a dose of 8 mg was optimal [96]. For augmentation of analgesia, a dose of 4 mg dexamethasone resulted in less inhibition of prostanoids and less effective analgesia after dental surgery than ketorolac 30 mg [97]. Bisgaard et al. [88] reported that an 8 mg dose of dexamethasone was sufficient for pain relief. Dexamethasone has also been tested for local application as an endo-alveolar powder or local infiltration in wisdom tooth surgery [98]. However, the dose used was 4–10 mg, and a systemic effect cannot be ruled out in this experimental design. In another dental surgery study, 8 mg dexamethasone was found to be more efficient than 4 mg, but increasing the dose to 16 mg did not provide any further improvement in pain relief [99]. The dose of gluco-corticoid used in the studies from Romundstad's group [79,89] is more generous, as the 125 mg methylprednisolone dose they employed is equivalent to 25 mg of dexamethasone [80]. Olstad also reported that 84 mg methylprednisolone administered over 4 days was effective for pain post dental surgery [100].

Although glucocorticoids have been shown to inhibit the cyclooxygenase II (COX-II) enzyme system, much like NSAIDs, they also have hormonal effects and act on a variety of other enzyme systems. Thus, it is of interest to elucidate how the analgesic effect compares with that of other analgesics in placebo-controlled models: Olstad studied the effect of betamethasone versus paracetamol over 4 days and found a tendency for paracetamol to be more analgesic during the 3–4 h after administration, whereas betamethasone was best during days 3 and 4 [100]. Romundstad et al. found that the analgesic effect of a single prophylactic 125 mg dose of methylprednisolone was equivalent to parecoxib 40 mg during a 6-h study period, with significantly less nausea and sedation [89]. These authors also evaluated the effectiveness of methylprednisolone 125 mg versus ketorolac 30 mg given for postoperative pain. They found that both drugs provided equivalent and effective analgesia during the first 24 h. Patients treated with ketorolac experienced a more rapid onset of analgesia, while those treated with methylprednisolone required significantly less rescue analgesic during postoperative days 2 and 3 [79].

An important question that must be answered is whether the glucocorticoids provide measurable analgesic effects when given alone, and whether they provide additive analgesic effects when administered with other analgesics [86,101,102].

In Bisgaard's study [88], the analgesic effect of dexamethasone 8 mg was in addition to a regimen of local wound anesthesia, paracetamol, and ketorolac. These analgesics were also given to the placebo patients. Similarly, in the study performed by Romundstad, the analgesic effect of a glucocorticoid was in addition to that provided by local anesthesia, paracetamol, and codeine [89]. Coloma supplied ketorolac and local anesthesia to all patients for baseline analgesia [87]. Several studies have been designed to test the specific analgesic effects of a glucocorticoid plus an NSAID or COX inhibitor. In one such study of pain post-dental surgery, Bamgbose et al. added dexamethasone 8 mg to diclofenac and reported improved pain score at 48 h with the combination [91]. In a similar clinical model, Moore et al. found that 10 mg dexamethasone added to rofecoxib 50 mg provided superior pain relief for up to 24 h than either drug administered alone [103]. Lin and coworkers [92] found that patients treated with the combination of 10 mg prednisolone plus diclofenac experienced significant reductions in gingival swelling following dental surgery [92]. In a study of dexamethasone 16 mg on top of rofecoxib and paracetamol, Hval et al. showed additional analgesic effects of dexamethasone [93].

Other clinical effects and side-effects

Glucocorticoids may also have beneficial effects on postoperative nausea and vomiting (PONV) [104,105], alertness, appetite, and mood [106]. Potential negative effects include hyperglycemia [107], flushing, restlessness, impaired wound healing, gastrointestinal ulceration, and increased infection risk [108]. Increased alertness has also been described [88,109] and may result in potential benefits in more rapid clearheaded recovery and discharge. Adverse effects are unlikely following single-dose administration but may increase with repeated doses [89,104, 109].

In a meta-analyses by Henzi et al. of the side-effects after single-dose administration, no significant side-effects were demonstrated in the 17 studies of 941 patients receiving dexamethasone [104]. Even more impressive is the absence of side-effects revealed in the meta-analyses of a much higher dose of methylprednisolone (i.e., 15–30 mg/kg) used for chest-trauma care [108]. In more than 2000 patients from 51 single studies, the only significant effect found was an improvement of pulmonary function with glucocorticoid [108]. However, there have been scattered reports of psychotic reactions after a single, high-dose administration of glucocorticoids [85,110]. Also, in a study of dexamethasone 10 mg, a mean 32% increase in postoperative blood sugar was noted, although no placebo group was included [107]. A recent concern arose from a study of dexamethasone for tonsillectomy where significantly more postoperative bleeding occurred after dexamethasone than placebo [111]. Still, as the bleeding numbers were low and the study design may be criticized, it may be too premature to abandon the very successful use of this single-dose technique in a lot of studies and routine praxis.

Conclusion, glucocorticoids

The glucocorticoids have postoperative analgesic effect with a delayed onset of 1–4 h and prolonged duration for at least 1–3 days after a single iv dose. The analgesic peak potency seems to be comparable to the effects provided by optimal doses of NSAIDs and paracetamol. The combination of a glucocorticoid plus NSAIDs provides additive anti-inflammatory effects and analgesia. In addition, the glucocorticoids may offer a safe and useful substitute for patients with known contraindications to NSAIDs (asthma, allergy, renal failure, bleeding tendency). My experience with nondiabetics is that I do not see any large increase in blood sugar (Doksroed, S; submitted). With diabetics the blood sugar may rise more, but this may be well controlled by adjusting subsequent insulin doses.

There seems to be no difference in the effects of different glucocorticoids, although very few comparative studies on equipotent doses of different drugs have been done. From a theoretical point of view, dexamethasone may be the most appropriate choice. This drug has no mineralocorticoid effect and has the most prolonged duration of effect after a single dose [80]. The optimal dose of dexamethasone that can be recommended remains unclear, and varies according to the location and severity of the surgery. With dexamethasone, reliable analgesic effects have been demonstrated with 8–16 mg after surgery of moderate invasiveness, however it remains to be determined whether higher doses may be more effective and more long lasting, especially since adverse events are minor even with very high doses [108]. There is great need for such studies to be done, and also for studies to test for the effects of glucocorticoids after major surgery, and for large-scale studies with better sensitivity and statistical power to test for any possible rare side-effects.

NMDA receptor antagonists

The NMDA receptor is a glutamate receptor characterized by affinity for N-methyl-D-aspartate. It has an allosteric binding site for the excitatory amino acid and a site within the channel itself to which magnesium ions bind in a voltage-dependent manner. The positive voltage dependence of channel conductance and the high permeability of the conducting channel to calcium ions are important in excitotoxicity and neuronal plasticity. Excitation of the NMDA receptor system in the dorsal horn plays an important role in the sensitization process [112]. The use of NMDA receptor antagonists has been shown to both prevent and reverse hyperalgesia in animal studies [113]. NMDA receptors have also been located in nonmyelinated axons in the periphery, thus indicating that excitatory amino acids, in addition to their role in the central nervous system, may play a role in primary nociception in the periphery [114]. The glutamate excitatory transmitter system is widespread in the central nervous system and is involved in many important physiological processes. NMDA receptor antagonism will therefore be prone to lead to unwanted side-effects, thus limiting its use in clinical pain treatment.

Ketamine, an anesthetic agent well known for more than 30 years, has been shown to interact with a number of receptor systems such as those for NMDA, opioids, monoamines, and muscarine [115]. In low doses it may result in selective, noncompetitive NMDA blockade [116]. Low doses of ketamine have in some studies been shown to have postoperative analgesic effects. Although most studies have focused on the use of ketamine for pre-emptive analgesia [117,118], some studies also advocate its use postoperatively [119]. There are, however, several studies that fail to show any effect of low-dose ketamine [120,121], especially when applied preoperatively in small doses. The use of larger doses of ketamine in the postoperative period is limited by its known psychomimetic side-effects. Analgesic concentrations of ketamine start at approximately 1–200 ng/ml, whereas plasma concentrations of ketamine on awakening from general anesthesia have been reported to be in the range of 6–1100 ng/ml. Psychedelic side-effects of ketamine are reported at plasma levels as low as 1–200 ng/ml [122].

Ketamine seems to have a potent analgesic effect on certain types of chronic pathologic pain conditions [123]. Studies on human volunteers seem to indicate that ketamine exerts its primary blocking effects when the NMDA-receptor-controlled ion channel has already been opened by a continuous nociceptive stimulus [124]. This could explain why ketamine is a poor analgesic when used pre-emptively or for acute pain, while it is highly efficacious for pathologic pain conditions. Ketamine has also been used as an epidural or intrathecal drug for pain alleviation after surgery. The efficacy of ketamine administered in these ways is controversial, and there are several reports of unpleasant systemic side-effects [125,126]. The neurotoxicity of spinal ketamine is not yet clear, and further animal studies are needed. There is an interaction between the NMDA receptor system and the opioid receptor system in the dorsal horn. Ketamine may be of benefit in combination with opioids, especially regarding the reduction of tolerance after long-term treatment with opioids [127,128].

Ketamine is a racemic mixture of two enantiomers, $S(+)$-ketamine and $R(-)$-ketamine. $S(+)$-ketamine is 3–4 times more potent than $R(-)$-ketamine. Although some report that the $S(+)$ enantiomer has fewer psychomimetic side-effects, there are clinical studies which indicate the opposite [129–131]. The $S(+)$ enantiomer is commercially available in some places in Europe, and further studies are necessary to establish whether the use of either one of the enantiomers has clinical advantages. In summary, the use of ketamine as an analgesic in the immediate postoperative period is of limited value. Other NMDA antagonists with a better specificity and affinity, such as dextromethorphan, may prove more beneficial and are now under clinical investigation [132].

Membrane-stabilizing drugs: antineuropathics

Calcium channel blockers: gabapentin and pregabalin

Pregabalin and gabapentin are GABA analogs with anti-epileptic, analgesic, and anxiolytic activities. Pregabalin was developed as a follow-up compound to gabapentin, and is the S-enantiomer of racemic 3-isobutyl GABA. Pregabalin has a more predictable dose–effect relationship, a more prolonged duration of effect, and an improved side-effect profile. Pregabalin has demonstrated efficacy at doses 2–4 times lower than gabapentin, and seems to have a higher affinity to the binding site at the α_2-δ-subunit. Pregabalin and gabapentin work by modulating the presynaptic release of excitatory neurotransmitters such as glutamate, substance P, and norepinephrine. They bind selectively to the α_2-δ-subunit of voltage-sensitive calcium channels [133]. The action of these compounds seems to be restricted to neurons and they have minor effects on blood pressure and heart rate, like the vascular calcium channel blockers [134]. Gabapentin and pregabalin modulate the release of sensory neuropeptides, but only under conditions corresponding to inflammation-induced sensitization of the spinal cord. Gabapentin has a well-established role in the treatment of chronic pain conditions [135], especially in neuropathic pain such as post-herpetic neuralgia and diabetic neuropathy [136]. Pregabalin has also been shown to be effective in alleviating pain in chronic, neuropathic pain conditions [137–139].

Pregabalin and gabapentin have been shown to have analgesic, antineuropathic, and opioid-sparing effects in acute pain. Although acute pain is predominately nociceptive in nature, prolonged central sensitization with some degree of hyperalgesia will occur following trauma, thus giving a rational reason for administering gabapentin and pregabalin in acute pain. Furthermore, surgical trauma commonly involves damage to small nerve fibers and neurons, which also explains the activity of these agents in acute pain and their potential efficacy during the initial development of neuropathic pain.

In a systematic review of randomized controlled trials, a single dose of gabapentin (1200 mg or less) given preoperatively significantly reduced pain intensity and opioid consumption for the first 24 h after surgery [140]. Time to first request for rescue analgesia was also prolonged in subgroups receiving 1200 mg. Multiple dosing preoperatively and/or continued use postoperatively did not reduce visual analog scores (VAS) further. Gabapentin also reduced postoperative pain and vomiting; the mechanism probably reflects the significant reduction in opioid consumption [140]. In a study of 1800 mg gabapentin alone or in combination with rofecoxib for 3 days after hysterectomy, the combination was superior to either of the drugs alone or placebo. However at this dose sedation was more frequent in the gabapentin groups [141].

Fewer studies have, so far, been published on acute pain treatment with pregabalin. In a molar extraction dental pain model, 300 mg pregabalin given after surgery significantly reduced postoperative pain as measured by pain relief and pain intensity difference. A 300 mg dose was more efficacious than 50 mg pregabalin. Pregabalin was comparable to ibuprofen 400 mg and significantly superior to placebo [142]. Side-effects such as dizziness, somnolence, and vomiting were more frequent in the 300 mg group.

In conclusion, a preoperative dose of either 1200 mg gabapentin or 150 mg pregabalin reduces postoperative pain intensity and opioid consumption with few side-effects. The reduction in opioid dose requirement might decrease associated side-effects such as nausea and vomiting. The combination of pregabalin plus NSAID seems advisable as it would block both the neuropathic and inflammatory components of acute pain [143]. Still more studies are needed in the ambulatory setting as both the sedative/hypnotic effect of these drugs and the potential for hypotension may be a specific concern when patients are sent home.

Sodium channel blockers: lidocaine, mexiletine

Sodium channels are universally located on neurons and nerve fibers, being responsible for the propagation of an action potential along the cell membrane. A complete and reversible block of these channels can stop the nerve impulse, which is thought to be the major mechanism for the common use of local anesthetics. For obvious reasons a complete and generalized sodium channel block, as may be accomplished by tetrodotoxin from the Japanese puffer fish, may be lethal. However, there are also sodium channels in the periphery that are resistant to this toxin, and these have been shown to be of importance in conditions of neuropathic pain [144]. Systemic low concentrations of lidocaine and the oral analog mexiletine act on these channels. They have been shown to be efficient analgesics in neuropathic pain syndromes, such as diabetic neuropathy [145] and reflex sympathetic dystrophy syndrome [146,147]. Action on receptors of the G-protein and NMDA types has been suggested as the analgesic mechanism of these drugs [148]. The prolonged analgesic effect is thought to be caused by inhibition of spontaneous impulse generation in injured nerves and ganglion neurons proximal to injured nerve segments.

Efforts to produce drugs that act more specifically on tetrodotoxin-resistant channels are ongoing [149], but to date clinical trials have not been published. However, there are some studies showing significant effects on postoperative pain from intravenous lidocaine administration [144,148,150,151]. Although the clinical analgesic effect seemed modest, it was significant, and opioid sparing when added with paracetamol and NSAID [148]. Two studies have shown that continuous infusion of lidocaine improves bowel function after surgery [144,152], and Kaba et al. [148] have recently shown that the use of systemic lidocaine facilitates acute rehabilitation after laparoscopic surgery. Nevertheless, many questions regarding the optimal use of these agents and this analgesic principle remain unanswered. For example, what is the optimal dose of lidocaine? What is the optimal timing and duration of infusion? Will other local anesthetics be good alternatives? What is the potential of using oral alternatives (i.e., mexiletine) instead or additionally? Will new, more specific, drugs have better clinical potential?

α2-Adrenergic receptor agonists

The α2 receptor agonists have sedative, anxiolytic, analgesic, and hemodynamic properties [101]. They decrease sympathetic tone and will attenuate the neuroendocrine and hemodynamic response to anesthesia and surgery. They reduce opioid and anesthetic requirements in the perioperative setting, and provide measurable analgesia. In humans, α2 adrenoceptors are located in the dorsal horn of the spinal cord and in several areas of the brain. There are at

121

least three different subtypes of α2 adrenergic receptor: 2A, 2B, and 2C. Different subtypes may mediate antinociception and sedation separately and be a target for further drug refinement in this class [153]. Sedation is one major effect or side-effect of α2 agonists, and dexmedetomidine has recently been approved by the Food and Drug Administration (FDA) for use as a sedative in intensive care units. For specific pain treatment the use of high doses of α2 agonists is limited by their sedative/anesthetic properties, probably by an action in the locus ceruleus. Sedation after epidural administration of clonidine reflects a substantial systemic absorption.

The current α2 agonists used in pain management are clonidine, tizanidine, dexmedetomidine, and epinephrine. These compounds have different partial agonist properties, dexmedetomidine with a selectivity ratio of 1600:1 for α2:α1; clonidine, 200:1; and epinephrine, 1:1. New agonists such as radolmidine with high α2 selectivity are currently being investigated in animal models. They have a better pharmacokinetic profile with less rapid distribution within the central nervous system and may have the potential to provide analgesia with fewer central nervous system side-effects [154].

Intrathecally administered α2 agonists produce antinociception in much lower doses than when administered systemically, thus indicating that the main site for analgesia is in the neuraxis [155]. Clonidine is used as a co-analgesic in neuraxial blockades [155]. When administered epidurally or intrathecally, α2 agonists have synergistic action with opioids. An epidural bolus administration of the combination of fentanyl and clonidine will reduce the analgesic dose of each component by approximately 60% [156]. Clonidine will also enhance and prolong the effect of local anesthesia intrathecally [157,158]. Epinephrine is widely used as an epidural adjunct for postoperative pain relief, the effect being known for more than 50 years [159]. A mixture of 1 µg/ml epinephrine, together with 2 mg/ml bupivacaine and 1 µg/ml fentanyl is well documented for synergistic epidural pain relief with a minor incidence of motor block or hemodynamic instability [160]. Dexmedetomidine and other agonists also have analgesic properties when administered systemically. Dexmedetomidine at dose ranges from 0.5 µg/kg iv to 2.5 µg/kg im or orally results in significant analgesia with few side-effects [5, 6]. Dexmedetomidine is also highly efficacious when administered intrathecally or epidurally in animal models, but its use spinally in humans is still experimental.

Local administration of α2 agonists at the site of trauma seems to have analgesic properties [161,162], possibly by a reduction in norepinephrine release at nerve terminal endings. There is also evidence of additional analgesia when added to local anesthesia in peripheral nerve blocks or intravenous regional anesthesia [155,163].

In acute pain treatment, the use of α2 receptor agonists either in low doses systemically or as an adjuvant epidurally or intrathecally is highly beneficial. Their synergistic action with opioids and local anesthesia will reduce the doses needed of each drug, thus reducing the possible side-effects. The development of less lipid-soluble agonists and a better understanding of the different subtypes of the α2 receptors will probably result in an extended use of selective α2 agonists.

Other analgesic adjuvants

Cannabinoids

The discovery of the cannabinoid receptors CB_1 and CB_2 and their endogenous ligands has resulted in extensive research and the development of several cannabinoid receptor agonists and antagonists. Numerous animal studies have demonstrated analgesic and anti-hyperalgesic properties of both plant-derived and synthetic cannabinoids. Cannabinoids produce anti-nociception in acute pain models in animals [164]. However, the number of clinical trials investigating their acute analgesic effect on humans is limited and the results are mixed. Nabilone, a synthetic cannabinoid, had no or a negative effect on pain scores in patients undergoing major surgery [165]. In a multicenter dose-escalation study, 10–15 mg of an oral cannabis extract (cannador) resulted in a dose-related reduction in rescue analgesia requirements in a postoperative pain model [166]. Buggy et al. found no effect of 5 mg tetrahydrocannabinol (THC) in a double-blinded, placebo-controlled study in women after hysterectomy [167]. Drowsiness and cardiovascular events such as tachycardia, bradycardia, and hypotension are known possible side-effects of cannabinoids [168]. In conclusion, further studies are needed in order to evaluate the possible beneficial role of cannabinoids in the acute pain setting.

Nicotine

As pain generation and mediation may be inhibited by acetylcholine action, there has been some interest in looking at the antinociceptive effect of different cholinergic agonists [169,170]. Nicotine is one potential agonist candidate, readily available in tablets and skin pads. It has been shown that regular nicotine users (i.e., smokers) may have more postoperative pain than nonsmokers [171,172], especially when they have to abstain from smoking [173]. In a study of uterine surgery, Flood and Daniel showed that a single dose of nasal nicotine just after the end of uterine surgery resulted in lower pain scores during the first postoperative 24 h, without any side-effects [174]. However, few studies have yet been done on nicotine analgesia in the clinical setting.

Neostigmine

Another way of producing analgesia is to enhance endogenous acetylcholine levels by using neostigmine [175]. Neostigmine is an inhibitor of the acetylcholinesterase enzyme, thus providing higher concentrations of acetylcholine in the synaptic area. A problem, limiting the exploitation of this analgesic mechanism, has been the high incidence of nausea that results from neostigmine's activity in the brainstem emesis center. Nausea is most prominent when neostigmine is given intrathecally, whereas epidural or peripheral administration is associated with a gradual dose–response curve for emetic side-effects [176]. Neostigmine provides useful analgesic effects with epidural or caudal routes of administration, whereas intra-articular and intravenous regional administration are associated with more conflicting results [176–179]. It has also been questioned whether there is any physiologic reason to believe in a role for acetylcholine in pain mechanisms outside the central nervous system [180], suggesting that any effect seen from topical administration may be a central one.

Magnesium

Magnesium ions normally "plug" the ion channels of NMDA receptors in the resting state. Dissociation of magnesium ions is believed to be a mandatory first step to activation of these receptors and enhances pain transmission and sensitization. Receptor antagonists, such as ketamine, block NMDA activation; however, another way to limit activity is to rapidly replace the magnesium-ion "lock" by having increased concentrations of magnesium in the extracellular environment. Indeed, there are numerous clinical studies showing that infusion of magnesium in the perioperative phase has an additive analgesic action [181–185]. There are several negative studies as well [186,187]. Positive effects have been demonstrated after various types of surgery: gynecologic, prostate, cardiac, ear, nose and throat, and cholecystectomy. Typically, 20–50 mg/kg magnesium sulfate is given slowly at the start of anesthesia, followed by an infusion of 10–20 mg/kg per hour for up to 1–3 days. In a dose-finding study Seyhan et al. found a 40 mg/kg bolus followed by infusion of 10 mg/kg per hour for 4 h to be the optimal dose, with no more analgesia gained by doubling the infusion rate [183]. Some studies have also shown prolonged (i.e., until next morning) postoperative efficacy by utilizing a single bolus dose, without the need for infusion [185,188]. Topical administration has also been shown to be safe and effective in patients recovering from knee surgery [189] and in intravenous regional anesthesia [190]. In one study looking specifically at magnesium in addition to ketamine for tonsillectomies, there was no analgesic effect of either drug, or of their combination [186].

Nonpharmacologic approaches

Nonpharmacologic measures may be valuable supplements in the treatment of acute pain. Acupuncture and transcutaneous electrical nerve stimulation (TENS) have been scientifically proven to provide analgesia, but will usually be a little too cumbersome and demanding for short-lasting pain after ambulatory surgery. Psychoprophylaxis, i.e., preoperative psychologic preparation for a surgical procedure, is also an interesting option in the nonpharmacologic approach to optimal pain treatment. Thorough communication of information, by both surgeon and anesthetist, about the surgical procedure, anesthesia technique, and pain treatment will reduce anxiety and stress. It has been known for decades that psychoprophylaxis reduces the need for postoperative analgesics [191]. In a more recent study, Doering et al. [192] investigated the use of the preoperative presentation of a videotape showing a patient undergoing total hip replacement surgery. This prophylactic procedure significantly reduced the perioperative anxiety level and the need for postoperative analgesic medication in patients undergoing hip surgery. Also in children, a preoperative video preparing for what is going to happen before and after surgery may be very useful.

The clinical application of nonopioids: putting it all together

Unlike opioids, most nonopioid analgesics and adjuvants have a maximal effect ceiling and a delayed onset of action. Further, as discussed, many of these drugs, especially local anesthetics, ketamine, NSAIDs/COX inhibitors, and glucocorticoids, may have a pre-emptive or at least preventive effect [1], thus there is a rationale to administer these agents as early as possible before or during exposure to trauma. In this section I will not include most of the "new" analgesic options described above. This is mainly due to a lack of extensive documentation of a clinically relevant effect in addition to that provided by established multimodal care, and due to incomplete documentation on optimal dosing and the risk of rare side-effects. These issues may change during the next few years. Also, there may be good reason to encourage clinicians to test out some of these modalities, especially in patients for whom standard opioid-based regimens prove to be suboptimal. Preferably, such testing should be done in controlled studies, in order to share reliable experiences with colleagues and also to contribute to the development of sound, scientific knowledge on the practical use of these agents.

I have included the glucocorticoids in our basic regimens, as I feel the documentation and clinical use here is adequate for making general recommendations. With ketamine, I think some dosing issues remain to be resolved. Apart from the fact that this drug should probably be given as an infusion for some time, the addition of extra labor and complexity to perioperative care has to be justified better in terms of clinical benefits. With the calcium blockers, systemic local anesthetics, and cannabinoids we think the documentation generally is too sparse at the moment to justify general recommendations.

Acute postoperative pain

The cornerstones will be paracetamol (acetaminophen) and NSAIDs/COX inhibitors for all patients, unless contraindicated, and local anesthesia whenever feasible in all wounds, and even better as dedicated nerve or plexus blocks.

Preoperatively

In order to ensure an empty stomach before anesthetic induction and also systemic absorption of the drug, paracetamol and a NSAID/COX inhibitor should be given orally at least 1 h ahead of surgery. Oral paracetamol should be administered as a 2 g dose for regular adults; for those with a body weight of less than 60 kg or those older than 70 years the dose should be reduced to 1.5 g. Paracetamol is also available in many places as a rapidly soluble tablet. There are data suggesting that rapidly soluble tablets allow a peak serum concentration to be reached as quickly as at 27 min after ingestion, compared with 45 min for ordinary tablets [193]. Rectal administration of paracetamol/acetaminophen should only be used in cases of noncompliance or inaccessibility of the oral or iv route. With rectal administration the serum concentration peaks at a lower level and more variably at 3–4 h after administration. For rectal use in children a starting dose of 50mg/kg is recommended.

NSAIDs, such as diclofenac (100 mg), naproxen (500 mg), or ibuprofen (800 mg), should also be given orally at least 1 h ahead of surgery; again dose reduction should be undertaken in small adults and the elderly above 70 years of age. In children, ibuprofen or diclofenac are licensed down to 1 year of age in many countries; the typical dose is 15–20 mg/kg (ibuprofen) or 1–2 mg/kg (diclofenac). As the COX-II inhibitors seem to carry no more cardiovascular risk than most traditional NSAIDs, such as diclofenac or ibuprofen, the threshold for using a COX-II inhibitor instead of NSAID should be rather low. As regulatory and medicolegal issues calm down after the strong actions taken after the Vioxx® case, we may have the COX-II inhibitors back as our preferred and routine alternative to NSAIDs preoperatively, because of their lack of effect on platelets and coagulation function. Until then, there may still be good reason to prefer the COX-II inhibitors: where there is fear of bleeding problems (should be discussed with the surgeon), in patients with a history of gastric ulcer problems, and in allergic or asthmatic patients. Celecoxib is well documented at a starting dose of 400 mg followed by 200 mg twice a day (bid). In Europe, etoricoxib is approved for use and a single dose of 120 mg can provide up to 24 h of safe and effective analgesia in uncompromised patients.

If oral medication preoperatively is not feasible or practical (e.g., too short a time delay before the start of anesthesia, gastric suction needed during surgery), the starting dose of iv paracetamol or NSAIDs, i.e., ketorolac (or parecoxib in the case of a COX-II inhibitor) may alternatively be given intravenously shortly after the induction of anesthesia. There are reasons to believe that the iv paracetamol starting dose should also be 2 g instead of the recommended 1 g dose commonly used. For ketorolac and parecoxib the starting doses will typically be 30 mg and 40 mg, respectively.

Peroperatively, early phase

After establishment of the iv line in the operating room, glucocorticoids are recommended to be administrated as early as possible due to their slow onset of clinical action. However, injection of the common solvent in the dexamethasone preparations may result in perineal and genital burning aching in patients, and this is not perceived as a good or appropriate experience prior to anesthetic induction. For this reason dexamethasone, in typical doses (8 mg for minor surgery, 16 mg for major surgery in adults, and 0.25–0.5 mg/kg in children), is best given after induction, or slowly injected after the start of sedation in awake patients receiving regional anesthesia. If the surgeon accepts the use of local anesthesia infiltration prior to the dissection in the surgical field, there is documentation as to the benefits of pre-emptive dosing, although not very strong [1]. Lidocaine 5–10 mg/ml has a rapid onset and with epinephrine added the duration is moderately prolonged and hemostasis is improved. Nevertheless, bupivacaine 2.5 mg/ml is the preferred agent for prolonged postoperative analgesia (up to 10–15 h). Care should always be taken to avoid high doses and systemic toxicity. If a dose of more than 40 ml (of the 2.5 ml/mg solution) is needed, the infiltration should be with the less toxic levobupivacaine (2.5 mg/ml) or ropivacaine (2–5mg/ml) instead.

If high doses of remifentanil are used, i.e., more than 0.3 μg/kg per minute or a plasma target of more than 7–8 ng/ml for more than 2–3 h, there are data suggesting the development of postoperative hyperalgesia by NMDA receptor activation. The best documented way of blocking this hyperalgesia is to employ a low-dose infusion of ketamine, i.e., 1–2 μg/kg per minute, peroperatively and for some hours postoperatively. There is also evidence to suggest that general anesthesia with potent inhalational agents or nitrous oxide will attenuate remifentanil hyperalgesia. Also perioperative administration of NSAIDs or COX inhibitors may blunt hyperalgesia [194].

Postoperatively in the PACU/hospital

In this phase there will be an iv line for drug administration and qualified nurses caring for the patients, thus allowing for their individualized care. Medication with paracetamol (1 g every 6 h in adults; 25–30 mg/kg every 6 h in children) and NSAID/COX inhibitor (prescription doses and intervals) should be used as baseline prophylactic medication. In the case of pain, an extra iv dose of ketorolac should be considered (see above). If parecoxib was given peroperatively a repeated dose may be considered after 4–6 h. When patients are still in pain, small, titrated doses of opioid should be added. Fentanyl 0.5–1 μg/kg is a good routine opioid, with a fairly rapid onset of action within 3–4 min and a limited duration of action (20–40 min after small doses), allowing for reduced risk of overdosing and subsequent nausea or somnolence. Recent evidence has suggested that oxycodone may be a better alternative for visceral pain, with better analgesia and less sedation than morphine [194]. This is due to either some action on the kappa receptors in addition to primary mu receptor effects, or faster penetration into the cerebrospinal cells.

Postoperatively at home or without iv access at hospital ward/hotel

Whereas glucocorticoids alone are recommended as a single dose peroperatively with a potential effect for 2–3 days, the dosing of paracetamol and NSAID/COX-II inhibitor should be repeated routinely as basic prophylactic medication at prescription doses throughout this phase. Typically, NSAIDs or COX-II inhibitors may be dosed for 1, 3, 5, or 10 days according to the expected duration of intermediate pain after the procedure in question, whereas paracetamol should be used for the whole period of postoperative pain, extending up to 1–2 weeks or more. If anything is needed on top for analgesia, oral oxycodone seems to be a well-absorbed and efficient alternative. The slow release formulation of 5, 10, or 20 mg may be used twice as basic medication, whereas the 5 or 10 mg routine formulation may be used as needed on top of this.

Table 6.1. A balanced approach to postoperative pain medication

Preoperatively:	Paracetamol 1.5–2 g orally (40–50 mg/kg children) COX-II inhibitor/NSAID orally
Perioperatively:	Local anesthesia as extensively as possible Dexamethasone 8 mg iv (paracetamol + NSAID/COX-II inhibitor if not given preoperatively)
Postoperatively, in hospital:	Fentanyl if needed Top-up dose of iv NSAID Continue paracetamol every 6 h
At home, phase I:	Paracetamol 1 g × 4 NSAID/COX-II inhibitor × 1–3 (depending on drug) If needed: oxycodone (fast or slow release) in addition
At home, phase II:	Paracetamol NSAID/COX-II inhibitor, if needed

Conclusions

The guiding principal is to reduce opioid dosing for acute pain as much as possible by using nonopioids and adjuvants in maximum tolerable doses, in a stepwise fashion, according to intensity of the pain stimulus. In a clinical context, single pre- or perioperative doses of glucocorticoid, paracetamol/acetaminophen should be considered and administered in appropriate patients. In combination with standardized regional analgesia, NSAIDs or COX-II inhibitors, and limited doses of opioid, the overall quality of pain management, rehabilitation, and return to functionality can be optimized while patient safety is maintained (Table 6.1).

References

1. Ong CK, Lirk P, Seymour RA, Jenkins BJ. The efficacy of preemptive analgesia for acute postoperative pain management: a meta-analysis. *Anesth Analg* 2005;**100**:757–73, table.

2. Myre KS, Raeder J, Rostrup M, et al. Catecholamine release during laparoscopic fundoplication with high and low doses of remifentanil. *Acta Anaesthesiol Scand* 2003;**47**:267–73.

3. Moss J, Rosow CE. Development of peripheral opioid antagonists; new insights into opioid effects. *Mayo Clin Proc* 2008;**83**:1116–30.

4. Tverskoy M, Cozacov C, Ayache M, et al. Postoperative pain after inguinal herniorrhaphy with different types of anesthesia. *Anesth Analg* 1990;**70**:29–35.

5. Moss G, Regal ME, Lichtig L. Reducing postoperative pain, narcotics, and length of hospitalization. *Surgery* 1986;**99**:206–10.

6. McLoughlin J, Kelley CJ. Study of the effectiveness of bupivacaine infiltration of the ilioinguinal nerve at the time of hernia repair for postoperative pain relief. *Br J Clin Pract* 1989;**43**:281–3.

7. Owen H, Galloway DJ, Mitchell KG. Analgesia by wound infiltration after surgical excision of benign breast lumps. *Ann R Coll Surg Engl* 1985;**67**:114–15.

8. Partridge BL, Stabile BE. The effects of incisional bupivacaine on postoperative narcotic requirements, oxygen saturation and length of stay in the post-anesthesia care unit. *Acta Anaesthesiol Scand* 1990;**34**:486–91.

9. Bourne MH, Johnson KA. Postoperative pain relief using local anesthetic instillation. *Foot Ankle* 1988;**8**:350–1.

10. Pryn SJ, Crosse MM, Murison MS, McGinn FP. Postoperative analgesia for haemorrhoidectomy. A comparison between caudal and local infiltration. *Anaesthesia* 1989;**44**:964–6.

11. Uzunkoy A, Coskun A, Akinci OF. The value of pre-emptive analgesia in the treatment of postoperative pain after laparoscopic cholecystectomy. *Eur Surg Res* 2001;**33**:39–41.

12. Sinclair R, Cassuto J, Hogstrom S, et al. Topical anesthesia with lidocaine aerosol in the control of postoperative pain. *Anesthesiology* 1988;**68**:895–901.

13. Narchi P, Benhamou D, Fernandez H. Intraperitoneal local anaesthetic for shoulder pain after day-case laparoscopy. *Lancet* 1991;**338**:1569–70.

14. Tree-Trakarn T, Pirayavaraporn S, Lertakyamanee J. Topical analgesia for relief of post-circumcision pain. *Anesthesiology* 1987;**67**:395–9.

15. Lisander B. An antiinflammatory effect of lidocaine? *Acta Anaesthesiol Scand* 1996;**40**:285–6.

16. Elhakim M, Elkott M, Ali NM, Tahoun HM. Intraperitoneal lidocaine for postoperative pain after laparoscopy. *Acta Anaesthesiol Scand* 2000;**44**:280–4.

17. Amid PK, Shulman AG, Lichtenstein IL. Local anesthesia for inguinal hernia repair step-by-step procedure. *Ann Surg* 1994;**220**:735–7.

18. Dahl JB, Moiniche S, Kehlet H. Wound infiltration with local anaesthetics for postoperative pain relief. *Acta Anaesthesiol Scand* 1994;**38**:7–14.

19. Renck H, Hassan HG, Lindberg B, Akerman B. Effects of macromolecular adjuvants on the duration of prilocaine. Experimental studies on the effect of variations of viscosity and sodium content and of inclusion of adrenaline. *Acta Anaesthesiol Scand* 1988;**32**:355–64.

20. Grant GJ, Lax J, Susser L, et al. Wound infiltration with liposomal bupivacaine prolongs analgesia in rats. *Acta Anaesthesiol Scand* 1997;**41**:204–7.

21. Dyhre H, Wallin R, Bjorkman S, et al. Inclusion of lignocaine base into a polar lipid formulation – in vitro release, duration of peripheral nerve block and arterial blood concentrations in the rat. *Acta Anaesthesiol Scand* 2001;**45**:583–9.

22. Bannwarth B, Netter P, Lapicque F, et al. Plasma and cerebrospinal fluid concentrations of paracetamol after a single intravenous dose of propacetamol. *Br J Clin Pharmacol* 1992;**34**:79–81.

23. Piletta P, Porchet HC, Dayer P. Central analgesic effect of acetaminophen but not of aspirin. *Clin Pharmacol Ther* 1991;**49**:350–4.

24. Broze GJ, Jr., Girard TJ, Novotny WF. The lipoprotein-associated coagulation inhibitor. *Prog Hemost Thromb* 1991;**10**:243–68.

25. Moore A, Collins S, Carroll D, McQuay H. Paracetamol with and without codeine in acute pain: a quantitative systematic review. *Pain* 1997;**70**:193–201.

26. Montgomery JE, Sutherland CJ, Kestin IG, Sneyd JR. Morphine consumption in patients receiving rectal paracetamol and diclofenac alone and in combination. *Br J Anaesth* 1996;**77**:445–7.

27. Seymour RA, Kelly PJ, Hawkesford JE. The efficacy of ketoprofen and paracetamol (acetaminophen) in postoperative pain after third molar surgery. *Br J Clin Pharmacol* 1996;**41**:581–5.

28. Breivik EK, Barkvoll P, Skovlund E. Combining diclofenac with acetaminophen or acetaminophen-codeine after oral surgery: a randomized, double-blind single-dose study. *Clin Pharmacol Ther* 1999;**66**:625–35.

29. Anderson BJ, Holford NH, Woollard GA, et al. Perioperative pharmacodynamics of acetaminophen analgesia in children. *Anesthesiology* 1999;**90**:411–21.

30. Korpela R, Korvenoja P, Meretoja OA. Morphine-sparing effect of acetaminophen in pediatric day-case surgery. *Anesthesiology* 1999;**91**:442–7.

31. Bremerich DH, Neidhart G, Heimann K, et al. Prophylactically administered rectal acetaminophen does not reduce

postoperative opioid requirements in infants and small children undergoing elective cleft palate repair. *Anesth Analg* 2001;**92**:907–12.

32. Blume H, Ali SL, Elze M, et al. [Relative bioavailability of paracetamol in suppository preparations in comparison to tablets.] *Arzneimittelforschung* 1994;**44**:1333–8.

33. Peduto VA, Ballabio M, Stefanini S. Efficacy of propacetamol in the treatment of postoperative pain. Morphine-sparing effect in orthopedic surgery. Italian Collaborative Group on Propacetamol. *Acta Anaesthesiol Scand* 1998;**42**:293–8.

34. Walson PD, Jones J, Chesney R, Rodarte A. Antipyretic efficacy and tolerability of a single intravenous dose of the acetaminophen prodrug propacetamol in children: a randomized, double-blind, placebo-controlled trial. *Clin Ther* 2006;**28**:762–9.

35. Duggan ST, Scott LJ. Intravenous paracetamol (acetaminophen). *Drugs* 2009;**69**:101–13.

36. Juhl GI, Norholt SE, Tonnesen E, et al. Analgesic efficacy and safety of intravenous paracetamol (acetaminophen) administered as a 2 g starting dose following third molar surgery. *Eur J Pain* 2006;**10**:371–7.

37. Rannug U, Holme JA, Hongslo JK, Sram R. International Commission for Protection against Environmental Mutagens and Carcinogens. An evaluation of the genetic toxicity of paracetamol. *Mutat Res* 1995;**327**:179–200.

38. Bach PH, Hardy TL. Relevance of animal models to analgesic-associated renal papillary necrosis in humans. *Kidney Int* 1985;**28**:605–13.

39. Peterson RG, Rumack BH. Age as a variable in acetaminophen overdose. *Arch Intern Med* 1981;**141**:390–3.

40. Bergman K, Muller L, Teigen SW. Series: current issues in mutagenesis and carcinogenesis, No. 65. The genotoxicity and carcinogenicity of paracetamol: a regulatory (re)view. *Mutat Res* 1996;**349**:263–88.

41. Girard P, Pansart Y, Coppe MC, et al. Modulation of paracetamol and nefopam antinociception by serotonin 5-HT(3) receptor antagonists in mice. *Pharmacology* 2009;**83**:243–6.

42. Vane JR. Inhibition of prostaglandin synthesis as a mechanism of action for aspirin-like drugs. *Nat New Biol* 1971;**231**:232–5.

43. Trang LE. Prostaglandins and inflammation. *Semin Arthritis Rheum* 1980;**9**:153–90.

44. Romsing J, Moiniche S, Ostergaard D, Dahl JB. Local infiltration with NSAIDs for postoperative analgesia: evidence for a peripheral analgesic action. *Acta Anaesthesiol Scand* 2000;**44**:672–83.

45. Bjorkman RL, Hedner T, Hallman KM, et al. Localization of the central antinociceptive effects of diclofenac in the rat. *Brain Res* 1992;**590**:66–73.

46. Dahl JB, Kehlet H. Non-steroidal anti-inflammatory drugs: rationale for use in severe postoperative pain. *Br J Anaesth* 1991;**66**:703–12.

47. Dahl V, Raeder JC, Drosdal S, et al. Prophylactic oral ibuprofen or ibuprofen-codeine versus placebo for postoperative pain after primary hip arthroplasty. *Acta Anaesthesiol Scand* 1995;**39**:323–6.

48. Sandhu DP, Iacovou JW, Fletcher MS, et al. A comparison of intramuscular ketorolac and pethidine in the alleviation of renal colic. *Br J Urol* 1994;**74**:690–3.

49. Bertin L, Pons G, d'Athis P, et al. A randomized, double-blind, multicentre controlled trial of ibuprofen versus acetaminophen and placebo for symptoms of acute otitis media in children. *Fundam Clin Pharmacol* 1996;**10**:387–92.

50. Mather SJ, Peutrell JM. Postoperative morphine requirements, nausea and vomiting following anaesthesia for tonsillectomy. Comparison of intravenous morphine and non-opioid analgesic techniques. *Paediatr Anaesth* 1995;**5**:185–8.

51. Bhatt-Mehta V, Rosen DA. Management of acute pain in children. *Clin Pharm* 1991;**10**:667–85.

52. Hawkey CJ. Non-steroidal anti-inflammatory drugs and peptic ulcers. *BMJ* 1990;**300**:278–84.

53. Strom BL, Berlin JA, Kinman JL, et al. Parenteral ketorolac and risk of gastrointestinal and operative site bleeding. A postmarketing surveillance study. *JAMA* 1996;**275**:376–82.

54. Feldman HI, Kinman JL, Berlin JA, et al. Parenteral ketorolac: the risk for acute renal failure. *Ann Intern Med* 1997;**126**:193–9.

55. Zikowski D, Hord AH, Haddox JD, Glascock J. Ketorolac-induced bronchospasm. *Anesth Analg* 1993;**76**:417–19.

56. Thwaites BK, Nigus DB, Bouska GW, et al. Intravenous ketorolac tromethamine does not worsen platelet function during knee arthroscopy under general anesthesia. *Anesth Analg* 1995;**81**:119–24.

57. Weale A, Warwick D, Durant N. Is there haemostatic interaction between low-molecular-weight heparin and non-steroidal analgesics after total hip replacement? *Lancet* 1993;**342**:995.

58. Goppelt-Struebe M. Regulation of prostaglandin endoperoxide synthase (cyclooxygenase) isozyme expression. *Prostaglandins Leukot Essent Fatty Acids* 1995;**52**:213–22.

59. Mitchell JA, Akarasereenont P, Thiemermann C, et al. Selectivity of nonsteroidal antiinflammatory drugs as inhibitors of constitutive and inducible cyclooxygenase. *Proc Natl Acad Sci USA* 1993;**90**:11693–7.

60. Zhu X, Conklin D, Eisenach JC. Cyclooxygenase-1 in the spinal cord plays an important role in postoperative pain. *Pain* 2003;**104**:15–23.

61. Lenz H, Raeder J. Comparison of etoricoxib vs. ketorolac in postoperative pain relief. *Acta Anaesthesiol Scand* 2008;**52**:1278–84.

62. Cannon CP, Curtis SP, FitzGerald GA, et al. Cardiovascular outcomes with etoricoxib and diclofenac in patients with osteoarthritis and rheumatoid arthritis in the Multinational Etoricoxib and Diclofenac Arthritis Long-term (MEDAL) programme: a randomised comparison. *Lancet* 2006;**368**:1771–81.

63. Nussmeier NA, Whelton AA, Brown MT, et al. Complications of the COX-2 inhibitors parecoxib and valdecoxib after cardiac surgery. *N Engl J Med* 2005;**352**:1081–91.

64. Nussmeier NA, Whelton AA, Brown MT, et al. Safety and efficacy of the cyclooxygenase-2 inhibitors parecoxib and valdecoxib after noncardiac surgery. *Anesthesiology* 2006;**104**:518–26.

65. Slappendel R, Weber EW, Benraad B, et al. Does ibuprofen increase perioperative blood loss during hip arthroplasty? *Eur J Anaesthesiol* 2002;**19**:829–31.

66. Moiniche S, Romsing J, Dahl JB, Tramer MR. Nonsteroidal antiinflammatory drugs and the risk of operative site bleeding after tonsillectomy: a quantitative systematic review. *Anesth Analg* 2003;**96**:68–77, table.

67. Vuolteenaho K, Moilanen T, Moilanen E. Non-steroidal anti-inflammatory drugs, cyclooxygenase-2 and the bone healing process. *Basic Clin Pharmacol Toxicol* 2008;**102**:10–14.

68. Glassman SD, Rose SM, Dimar JR, et al. The effect of postoperative nonsteroidal anti-inflammatory drug administration on spinal fusion. *Spine (Phila Pa 1976)* 1998;**23**:834–8.

69. Buchman AL. Side effects of corticosteroid therapy. *J Clin Gastroenterol* 2001;**33**:289–94.

70. Skjelbred P, Lokken P. Post-operative pain and inflammatory reaction reduced by injection of a corticosteroid. A controlled trial in bilateral oral surgery. *Eur J Clin Pharmacol* 1982;**21**:391–6.

71. Holte K, Kehlet H. Perioperative single-dose glucocorticoid administration: pathophysiologic effects and clinical implications. *J Am Coll Surg* 2002;**195**:694–712.

72. Zhang RX, Lao L, Qiao JT, et al. Endogenous and exogenous glucocorticoid suppresses up-regulation of preprodynorphin mRNA and hyperalgesia in rats with peripheral inflammation. *Neurosci Lett* 2004;**359**:85–8.

73. Dallman MF. Fast glucocorticoid actions on brain: back to the future. *Front Neuroendocrinol* 2005;**26**:103–8.

74. Barnes PJ. Molecular mechanisms and cellular effects of glucocorticosteroids.

Immunol Allergy Clin North Am 2005;**25**:451–68.

75. Falkenstein E, Tillmann HC, Christ M, et al. Multiple actions of steroid hormones – a focus on rapid, nongenomic effects. *Pharmacol Rev* 2000;**52**:513–56.

76. Song IH, Buttgereit F. Non-genomic glucocorticoid effects to provide the basis for new drug developments. *Mol Cell Endocrinol* 2006;**246**:142–6.

77. Aasboe V, Raeder JC, Groegaard B. Betamethasone reduces postoperative pain and nausea after ambulatory surgery. *Anesth Analg* 1998;**87**:319–23.

78. Coloma M, White PF, Markowitz SD, et al. Dexamethasone in combination with dolasetron for prophylaxis in the ambulatory setting: effect on outcome after laparoscopic cholecystectomy. *Anesthesiology* 2002;**96**:1346–50.

79. Romundstad L, Breivik H, Niemi G, et al. Methylprednisolone intravenously 1 day after surgery has sustained analgesic and opioid-sparing effects. *Acta Anaesthesiol Scand* 2004;**48**:1223–31.

80. Salerno A, Hermann R. Efficacy and safety of steroid use for postoperative pain relief. Update and review of the medical literature. *J Bone Joint Surg Am* 2006;**88**:1361–72.

81. Hans P, Vanthuyne A, Dewandre PY, et al. Blood glucose concentration profile after 10 mg dexamethasone in non-diabetic and type 2 diabetic patients undergoing abdominal surgery. *Br J Anaesth* 2006;**97**:164–70.

82. O'Banion MK, Winn VD, Young DA. cDNA cloning and functional activity of a glucocorticoid-regulated inflammatory cyclooxygenase. *Proc Natl Acad Sci USA* 1992;**89**:4888–92.

83. Apfel CC, Korttila K, Abdalla M, et al. A factorial trial of six interventions for the prevention of postoperative nausea and vomiting. *N Engl J Med* 2004;**350**:2441–51.

84. Halvorsen P, Raeder J, White PF, et al. The effect of dexamethasone on side effects after coronary revascularization procedures. *Anesth Analg* 2003;**96**:1578–83, table.

85. Fleming PS, Flood TR. Steroid-induced psychosis complicating orthognathic

surgery: a case report. *Br Dent J* 2005;**199**:647–8.

86. White PF. The role of non-opioid analgesic techniques in the management of pain after ambulatory surgery. *Anesth Analg* 2002;**94**:577–85.

87. Coloma M, Duffy LL, White PF, et al. Dexamethasone facilitates discharge after outpatient anorectal surgery. *Anesth Analg* 2001;**92**:85–8.

88. Bisgaard T, Klarskov B, Kehlet H, Rosenberg J. Preoperative dexamethasone improves surgical outcome after laparoscopic cholecystectomy: a randomized double-blind placebo-controlled trial. *Ann Surg* 2003;**238**:651–60.

89. Romundstad L, Breivik H, Roald H, et al. Methylprednisolone reduces pain, emesis, and fatigue after breast augmentation surgery: a single-dose, randomized, parallel-group study with methylprednisolone 125 mg, parecoxib 40 mg, and placebo. *Anesth Analg* 2006;**102**:418–25.

90. Afman CE, Welge JA, Steward DL. Steroids for post-tonsillectomy pain reduction: meta-analysis of randomized controlled trials. *Otolaryngol Head Neck Surg* 2006;**134**:181–6.

91. Bamgbose BO, Akinwande JA, Adeyemo WL, et al. Effects of co-administered dexamethasone and diclofenac potassium on pain, swelling and trismus following third molar surgery. *Head Face Med* 2005;**1**:11.

92. Lin TC, Lui MT, Chang RC. Premedication with diclofenac and prednisolone to prevent postoperative pain and swelling after third molar removal. *Zhonghua Yi Xue Za Zhi (Taipei)* 1996;**58**:40–4.

93. Hval K, Thagaard KS, Schlichtihg E, Raeder J. The prolonged postoperative analgesic effect when dexamethasone is added to a nonsteroidal antiinflammatory drug before breast surgery. *Anesth Analg* 2007;**105**:481–6.

94. O'Sullivan BT, Cutler DJ, Hunt GE, et al. Pharmacokinetics of dexamethasone and its relationship to dexamethasone suppression test outcome in depressed patients and healthy control subjects. *Biol Psychiatry* 1997;**41**:574–84.

95. Liu K, Hsu CC, Chia YY. The effect of dose of dexamethasone for antiemesis after major gynecological surgery. *Anesth Analg* 1999;**89**:1316–18.

96. Lee Y, Lai HY, Lin PC, et al. A dose ranging study of dexamethasone for preventing patient-controlled analgesia-related nausea and vomiting: a comparison of droperidol with saline. *Anesth Analg* 2004;**98**:1066–71, table.

97. Dionne RA, Gordon SM, Rowan J, et al. Dexamethasone suppresses peripheral prostanoid levels without analgesia in a clinical model of acute inflammation. *J Oral Maxillofac Surg* 2003;**61**:997–1003.

98. Graziani F, D'Aiuto F, Arduino PG, et al. Perioperative dexamethasone reduces post-surgical sequelae of wisdom tooth removal. A split-mouth randomized double-masked clinical trial. *Int J Oral Maxillofac Surg* 2006;**35**:241–6.

99. Numazaki M, Fujii Y. Reduction of postoperative emetic episodes and analgesic requirements with dexamethasone in patients scheduled for dental surgery. *J Clin Anesth* 2005;**17**:182–6.

100. Olstad OA, Skjelbred P. Comparison of the analgesic effect of a corticosteroid and paracetamol in patients with pain after oral surgery. *Br J Clin Pharmacol* 1986;**22**:437–42.

101. Dahl V, Raeder JC. Non-opioid postoperative analgesia. *Acta Anaesthesiol Scand* 2000;**44**:1191–203.

102. Kehlet H, Jensen TS, Woolf CJ. Persistent postsurgical pain: risk factors and prevention. *Lancet* 2006;**367**:1618–25.

103. Moore PA, Brar P, Smiga ER, Costello BJ. Preemptive rofecoxib and dexamethasone for prevention of pain and trismus following third molar surgery. *Oral Surg Oral Med Oral Pathol Oral Radiol Endod* 2005;**99**:E1–E7.

104. Henzi I, Walder B, Tramer MR. Dexamethasone for the prevention of postoperative nausea and vomiting: a quantitative systematic review. *Anesth Analg* 2000;**90**:186–94.

105. Apfel CC, Korttila K, Abdalla M, et al. A factorial trial of six interventions for the prevention of postoperative nausea and vomiting. *N Engl J Med* 2004;**350**:2441–51.

106. Halvorsen P, Raeder J, White PF, et al. The effect of dexamethasone on side effects after coronary revascularization procedures. *Anesth Analg* 2003;**96**:1578–83, table.

107. Hans P, Vanthuyne A, Dewandre PY, et al. Blood glucose concentration profile after 10 mg dexamethasone in non-diabetic and type 2 diabetic patients undergoing abdominal surgery. *Br J Anaesth* 2006;**97**:164–70.

108. Sauerland S, Nagelschmidt M, Mallmann P, Neugebauer EA. Risks and benefits of preoperative high dose methylprednisolone in surgical patients: a systematic review. *Drug Saf* 2000;**23**:449–61.

109. Ahn JH, Kim MR, Kim KH. Effect of i.v. dexamethasone on postoperative dizziness, nausea and pain during canal wall-up mastoidectomy. *Acta Otolaryngol* 2005;**125**:1176–9.

110. Ferris RL, Eisele DW. Steroid psychosis after head and neck surgery: case report and review of the literature. *Otolaryngol Head Neck Surg* 2003;**129**:591–2.

111. Czarnetzki C, Elia N, Lysakowski C, et al. Dexamethasone and risk of nausea and vomiting and postoperative bleeding after tonsillectomy in children: a randomized trial. *JAMA* 2008;**300**:2621–30.

112. Woolf CJ, Thompson SW. The induction and maintenance of central sensitization is dependent on N-methyl-D-aspartic acid receptor activation; implications for the treatment of post-injury pain hypersensitivity states. *Pain* 1991;**44**:293–9.

113. Ma QP, Woolf CJ. Noxious stimuli induce an N-methyl-D-aspartate receptor-dependent hypersensitivity of the flexion withdrawal reflex to touch: implications for the treatment of mechanical allodynia. *Pain* 1995;**61**:383–90.

114. Carlton SM. Peripheral NMDA receptors revisited – hope floats. *Pain* 2009;**146**:1–2.

115. Hirota K, Lambert DG. Ketamine: its mechanism(s) of action and unusual clinical uses. *Br J Anaesth* 1996;**77**:441–4.

116. Eide PK, Stubhaug A, Breivik H, Oye I. Reply to S.T. Meller: Ketamine: relief from chronic pain through actions at the NMDA receptor. *Pain* 1997;**72**:289–91.

117. Tverskoy M, Oz Y, Isakson A, et al. Preemptive effect of fentanyl and ketamine on postoperative pain and wound hyperalgesia. *Anesth Analg* 1994;**78**:205–9.

118. Fu ES, Miguel R, Scharf JE. Preemptive ketamine decreases postoperative narcotic requirements in patients undergoing abdominal surgery. *Anesth Analg* 1997;**84**:1086–90.

119. Dich-Nielsen JO, Svendsen LB, Berthelsen P. Intramuscular low-dose ketamine versus pethidine for postoperative pain treatment after thoracic surgery. *Acta Anaesthesiol Scand* 1992;**36**:583–7.

120. Mathisen LC, Aasbo V, Raeder J. Lack of pre-emptive analgesic effect of (R)-ketamine in laparoscopic cholecystectomy. *Acta Anaesthesiol Scand* 1999;**43**:220–4.

121. Adam F, Libier M, Oszustowicz T, et al. Preoperative small-dose ketamine has no preemptive analgesic effect in patients undergoing total mastectomy. *Anesth Analg* 1999;**89**:444–7.

122. Bowdle TA, Radant AD, Cowley DS, et al. Psychedelic effects of ketamine in healthy volunteers: relationship to steady-state plasma concentrations. *Anesthesiology* 1998;**88**:82–8.

123. Eide PK, Jorum E, Stubhaug A, et al. Relief of post-herpetic neuralgia with the N-methyl-D-aspartic acid receptor antagonist ketamine: a double-blind, cross-over comparison with morphine and placebo. *Pain* 1994;**58**:347–54.

124. Arendt-Nielsen L, Petersen-Felix S, Fischer M, et al. The effect of N-methyl-D-aspartate antagonist (ketamine) on single and repeated nociceptive stimuli: a placebo-controlled experimental human study. *Anesth Analg* 1995;**81**:63–8.

125. Schneider I, Diltoer M. Continuous epidural infusion of ketamine during labour. *Can J Anaesth* 1987;**34**:657–8.

126. Bion JF. Intrathecal ketamine for war surgery. A preliminary study under field conditions. *Anaesthesia* 1984;**39**:1023–8.

127. Dickenson AH. NMDA receptor antagonists: interactions with opioids. *Acta Anaesthesiol Scand* 1997;**41**:112–15.

128. Bell RF. Low-dose subcutaneous ketamine infusion and morphine tolerance. *Pain* 1999;**83**:101–3.

129. White PF, Ham J, Way WL, Trevor AJ. Pharmacology of ketamine isomers in surgical patients. *Anesthesiology* 1980;**52**:231–9.

130. Calvey TN. Chirality in anaesthesia. *Anaesthesia* 1992;**47**:93–4.

131. Mathisen LC, Skjelbred P, Skoglund LA, Oye I. Effect of ketamine, an NMDA receptor inhibitor, in acute and chronic orofacial pain. *Pain* 1995;**61**:215–20.

132. Wu CT, Yu JC, Yeh CC, et al. Preincisional dextromethorphan treatment decreases postoperative pain and opioid requirement after laparoscopic cholecystectomy. *Anesth Analg* 1999;**88**:1331–4.

133. Zareba G. Pregabalin: a new agent for the treatment of neuropathic pain. *Drugs Today (Barc)* 2005;**41**:509–16.

134. Fink K, Dooley DJ, Meder WP, et al. Inhibition of neuronal Ca(2+) influx by gabapentin and pregabalin in the human neocortex. *Neuropharmacology* 2002;**42**:229–36.

135. Fehrenbacher JC, Taylor CP, Vasko MR. Pregabalin and gabapentin reduce release of substance P and CGRP from rat spinal tissues only after inflammation or activation of protein kinase C. *Pain* 2003;**105**:133–41.

136. Wiffen PJ, McQuay HJ, Edwards JE, Moore RA. Gabapentin for acute and chronic pain. *Cochrane Database Syst Rev* 2005; CD005452.

137. Bennett MI, Simpson KH. Gabapentin in the treatment of neuropathic pain. *Palliat Med* 2004;**18**:5–11.

138. Dworkin RH, Corbin AE, Young JP, Jr., et al. Pregabalin for the treatment of postherpetic neuralgia: a randomized, placebo-controlled trial. *Neurology* 2003;**60**:1274–83.

139. Freynhagen R, Strojek K, Griesing T, et al. Efficacy of pregabalin in neuropathic pain

evaluated in a 12-week, randomised, double-blind, multicentre, placebo-controlled trial of flexible- and fixed-dose regimens. *Pain* 2005;**115**:254–63.

140. Ho KY, Gan TJ, Habib AS. Gabapentin and postoperative pain – a systematic review of randomized controlled trials. *Pain* 2006;**126**:91–101.

141. Gilron I, Orr E, Tu D, et al. A placebo-controlled randomized clinical trial of perioperative administration of gabapentin, rofecoxib and their combination for spontaneous and movement-evoked pain after abdominal hysterectomy. *Pain* 2005;**113**:191–200.

142. Hill CM, Balkenohl M, Thomas DW, et al. Pregabalin in patients with postoperative dental pain. *Eur J Pain* 2001;**5**:119–24.

143. Reuben SS, Buvanendran A, Kroin JS, Raghunathan K. The analgesic efficacy of celecoxib, pregabalin, and their combination for spinal fusion surgery. *Anesth Analg* 2006;**103**:1271–7.

144. Groudine SB, Fisher HA, Kaufman RP, Jr., et al. Intravenous lidocaine speeds the return of bowel function, decreases postoperative pain, and shortens hospital stay in patients undergoing radical retropubic prostatectomy. *Anesth Analg* 1998;**86**:235–9.

145. Jarvis B, Coukell AJ. Mexiletine. A review of its therapeutic use in painful diabetic neuropathy. *Drugs* 1998;**56**:691–707.

146. Challapalli V, Tremont-Lukats IW, McNicol ED, et al. Systemic administration of local anesthetic agents to relieve neuropathic pain. *Cochrane Database Syst Rev* 2005;CD003345.

147. Kalso E. Sodium channel blockers in neuropathic pain. *Curr Pharm Des* 2005;**11**:3005–11.

148. Kaba A, Laurent SR, Detroz BJ, et al. Intravenous lidocaine infusion facilitates acute rehabilitation after laparoscopic colectomy. *Anesthesiology* 2007;**106**:11–18.

149. Akada Y, Ogawa S, Amano K, et al. Potent analgesic effects of a putative sodium channel blocker M58373 on formalin-induced and neuropathic pain in rats. *Eur J Pharmacol* 2006;**536**:248–55.

150. Koppert W, Weigand M, Neumann F, et al. Perioperative intravenous lidocaine has preventive effects on postoperative pain and morphine consumption after major abdominal surgery. *Anesth Analg* 2004;**98**:1050–5, table.

151. Fassoulaki A, Patris K, Sarantopoulos C, Hogan Q. The analgesic effect of gabapentin and mexiletine after breast surgery for cancer. *Anesth Analg* 2002;**95**:985–91, table.

152. Rimback G, Cassuto J, Tollesson PO. Treatment of postoperative paralytic ileus by intravenous lidocaine infusion. *Anesth Analg* 1990;**70**:414–19.

153. Buerkle H, Yaksh TL. Pharmacological evidence for different alpha 2-adrenergic receptor sites mediating analgesia and sedation in the rat. *Br J Anaesth* 1998;**81**:208–15.

154. Xu M, Kontinen VK, Kalso E. Effects of radolmidine, a novel alpha2 adrenergic agonist compared with dexmedetomidine in different pain models in the rat. *Anesthesiology* 2000;**93**:473–81.

155. Singelyn FJ, Dangoisse M, Bartholomee S, Gouverneur JM. Adding clonidine to mepivacaine prolongs the duration of anesthesia and analgesia after axillary brachial plexus block. *Reg Anesth* 1992;**17**:148–50.

156. Eisenach JC, D'Angelo R, Taylor C, Hood DD. An isobolographic study of epidural clonidine and fentanyl after cesarean section. *Anesth Analg* 1994;**79**:285–90.

157. Bonnet F, Brun-Buisson V, Saada M, et al. Dose-related prolongation of hyperbaric tetracaine spinal anesthesia by clonidine in humans. *Anesth Analg* 1989;**68**:619–22.

158. Liu S, Chiu AA, Neal JM, et al. Oral clonidine prolongs lidocaine spinal anesthesia in human volunteers. *Anesthesiology* 1995;**82**:1353–9.

159. Priddle HD, Andros GJ. Primary spinal anesthetic effects of epinephrine. *Curr Res Anesth Analg* 1950;**29**:156–62.

160. Niemi G, Breivik H. Adrenaline markedly improves thoracic epidural analgesia produced by a low-dose infusion of bupivacaine, fentanyl and adrenaline after

major surgery. A randomised, double-blind, cross-over study with and without adrenaline. *Acta Anaesthesiol Scand* 1998;**42**:897–909.

161. Davis KD, Treede RD, Raja SN, et al. Topical application of clonidine relieves hyperalgesia in patients with sympathetically maintained pain. *Pain* 1991;**47**:309–17.

162. Gentili M, Juhel A, Bonnet F. Peripheral analgesic effect of intra-articular clonidine. *Pain* 1996;**64**:593–6.

163. Memis D, Turan A, Karamanlioglu B, et al. Adding dexmedetomidine to lidocaine for intravenous regional anesthesia. *Anesth Analg* 2004;**98**:835–40, table.

164. Pertwee RG. Cannabinoid receptors and pain. *Prog Neurobiol* 2001;**63**:569–611.

165. Beaulieu P. Effects of nabilone, a synthetic cannabinoid, on postoperative pain. *Can J Anaesth* 2006;**53**:769–75.

166. Holdcroft A, Maze M, Dore C, et al. A multicenter dose-escalation study of the analgesic and adverse effects of an oral cannabis extract (Cannador) for postoperative pain management. *Anesthesiology* 2006;**104**:1040–6.

167. Buggy DJ, Toogood L, Maric S, et al. Lack of analgesic efficacy of oral delta-9-tetrahydrocannabinol in postoperative pain. *Pain* 2003;**106**:169–72.

168. Notcutt W, Price M, Miller R, et al. Initial experiences with medicinal extracts of cannabis for chronic pain: results from 34 'N of 1' studies. *Anaesthesia* 2004;**59**:440–52.

169. Decker MW, Rueter LE, Bitner RS. Nicotinic acetylcholine receptor agonists: a potential new class of analgesics. *Curr Top Med Chem* 2004;**4**:369–84.

170. Vincler M. Neuronal nicotinic receptors as targets for novel analgesics. *Expert Opin Investig Drugs* 2005;**14**:1191–8.

171. Creekmore FM, Lugo RA, Weiland KJ. Postoperative opiate analgesia requirements of smokers and nonsmokers. *Ann Pharmacother* 2004;**38**:949–53.

172. Woodside JR. Female smokers have increased postoperative narcotic requirements. *J Addict Dis* 2000;**19**:1–10.

173. Marco AP, Greenwald MK, Higgins MS. A preliminary study of 24-hour post-cesarean patient controlled analgesia: postoperative pain reports and morphine requests/utilization are greater in abstaining smokers than non-smokers. *Med Sci Monit* 2005;**11**: CR255–CR261.

174. Flood P, Daniel D. Intranasal nicotine for postoperative pain treatment. *Anesthesiology* 2004;**101**:1417–21.

175. Eisenach JC. Muscarinic-mediated analgesia. *Life Sci* 1999;**64**:549–54.

176. Habib AS, Gan TJ. Use of neostigmine in the management of acute postoperative pain and labour pain: a review. *CNS Drugs* 2006;**20**:821–39.

177. Gentili M, Enel D, Szymskiewicz O, et al. Postoperative analgesia by intraarticular clonidine and neostigmine in patients undergoing knee arthroscopy. *Reg Anesth Pain Med* 2001;**26**:342–7.

178. McCartney CJ, Brill S, Rawson R, et al. No anesthetic or analgesic benefit of neostigmine 1 mg added to intravenous regional anesthesia with lidocaine 0.5% for hand surgery. *Reg Anesth Pain Med* 2003;**28**:414–17.

179. Alagol A, Calpur OU, Usar PS, et al. Intraarticular analgesia after arthroscopic knee surgery: comparison of neostigmine, clonidine, tenoxicam, morphine and bupivacaine. *Knee Surg Sports Traumatol Arthrosc* 2005;**13**:658–63.

180. Schafer M. Analgesic effects of neostigmine in the periphery. *Anesthesiology* 2000;**92**:1207–8.

181. Tramer MR, Schneider J, Marti RA, Rifat K. Role of magnesium sulfate in postoperative analgesia. *Anesthesiology* 1996;**84**:340–7.

182. Bhatia A, Kashyap L, Pawar DK, Trikha A. Effect of intraoperative magnesium infusion on perioperative analgesia in open cholecystectomy. *J Clin Anesth* 2004;**16**:262–5.

183. Seyhan TO, Tugrul M, Sungur MO, et al. Effects of three different dose regimens of magnesium on propofol requirements, haemodynamic variables and postoperative

pain relief in gynaecological surgery. *Br J Anaesth* 2006;**96**:247–52.

184. Steinlechner B, Dworschak M, Birkenberg B, et al. Magnesium moderately decreases remifentanil dosage required for pain management after cardiac surgery. *Br J Anaesth* 2006;**96**:444–9.

185. Tauzin-Fin P, Sesay M, ort-Laval S, et al. Intravenous magnesium sulphate decreases postoperative tramadol requirement after radical prostatectomy. *Eur J Anaesthesiol* 2006;**23**:1055–9.

186. O'Flaherty JE, Lin CX. Does ketamine or magnesium affect posttonsillectomy pain in children? *Paediatr Anaesth* 2003;**13**:413–21.

187. Paech MJ, Magann EF, Doherty DA, et al. Does magnesium sulfate reduce the short- and long-term requirements for pain relief after caesarean delivery? A double-blind placebo-controlled trial. *Am J Obstet Gynecol* 2006;**194**:1596–602.

188. Levaux C, Bonhomme V, Dewandre PY, et al. Effect of intra-operative magnesium sulphate on pain relief and patient comfort after major lumbar orthopedic surgery. *Anaesthesia* 2003;**58**:131–5.

189. Bondok RS, bd El-Hady AM. Intra-articular magnesium is effective for postoperative analgesia in arthroscopic knee surgery. *Br J Anaesth* 2006;**97**:389–92.

190. Turan A, Memis D, Karamanlioglu B, et al. Intravenous regional anesthesia using lidocaine and magnesium. *Anesth Analg* 2005;**100**:1189–92.

191. Egbert LD, Battit GE, Welch CE, Bartlett MK. Reduction of postoperative pain by encouragement and instruction of patients. A study of doctor–patient rapport. *N Engl J Med* 1964;**270**:825–7.

192. Doering S, Katzlberger F, Rumpold G, et al. Videotape preparation of patients before hip replacement surgery reduces stress. *Psychosom Med* 2000;**62**:365–73.

193. Rygnestad T, Zahlsen K, Samdal FA. Absorption of effervescent paracetamol tablets relative to ordinary paracetamol tablets in healthy volunteers. *Eur J Clin Pharmacol* 2000;**56**:141–3.

194. Lenz H, Sandvik L, Qvigstad E, Bjerkelund CE, Raeder J. A comparison of intravenous oxycodone and intravenous morphine in patient-controlled postoperative analgesia after laparoscopic hysterectomy. *Anesth Analg.* 2009;**109**:1279–83.

Anti-emetic prophylaxis and treatment

Apart from postoperative pain, nausea and vomiting are the most frequent and disturbing side-effects experienced after ambulatory anesthesia [1], the reported incidence varying from almost zero [2] to 80% of the cases [3]. Even though the condition very rarely implies any danger of permanent sequelae and subsides spontaneously with time, it is nevertheless a frequent cause of delayed discharge, unplanned admission, extra work load and costs, dehydration, and considerable patient distress.

Nausea is defined as a subjective discomfort associated with the anticipation of retching or vomiting. Vomiting is the forceful expulsion of gastric contents and retching is similar to vomiting but occurs when there are no stomach contents expelled.

Although subjective feelings and their conscious manipulation are involved, vomiting and retching may be considered as objective outcomes. Nausea however is a subjective experience, which may be difficult to sort out in children and in patients with communication difficulties. In adults, nausea may also be complicated and enforced by other unpleasant sensations such as pain and anxiety. Nausea and vomiting are physiologic reflexes that are there to protect us from ingestion of poisonous food and fluids. Either receptors within the wall of the gut and stomach are activated by chemical stimuli or stretch, or poisonous molecules are absorbed into the blood and reach sensitive cells in the midbrain, which are then activated to initiate the feeling of nausea or the more complex neuromuscular reflex of retching or vomiting. Vestibular, visual or other types of brain nerve stimulation may also evoke nausea or vomiting. The conditions are closely linked: intense nausea will usually be accompanied by episodes of retching or vomiting, and vomiting will usually be preceded by nausea. However, there are examples of sudden, short-lasting vomiting with barely any nausea before or after the episode.

Physiology and anatomy

Nausea and vomiting are coordinated from an area close to the fourth ventricle (Figure 6.6) where the vessels are devoid of extra surrounding fat which otherwise constitutes the blood–brain barrier. Thus, the cells in this chemoreceptor zone are easily exposed to toxins diffusing from the blood. Most of the brain nerves have an input to this area, including the optical nerves, the vestibular (balance) nerve, and the vagal nerve (which receives input from the whole gastrointestinal system). A simplified view is that when the sum of input from brain nerves and firing in the chemoreceptor zone reaches a certain threshold, the result is output in terms of nausea and/or vomiting initiated in the nearby vomiting center. The level of this threshold varies considerably from person to person (Figure 6.7).

The principles of PONV prophylaxis and treatment address the reduction of incoming stimuli from the periphery and the resultant activation of receptors and cells in this midbrain area.

Etiology and risk factors [4–6]

The etiological factors may be divided into aspects associated with the patient, with the type of surgery, and with method of anesthesia and use of perioperative drugs (Table 6.2).

It has been shown that women of fertile age have a higher incidence of PONV than men, and furthermore that there is a modestly declining incidence with increasing age. Nonsmokers have a higher incidence than smokers, potentially because the latter's regular exposure to the toxins in smoke induces a degree of cellular adaptation; smoke in the naive nonsmoker can sometimes cause nausea. Individual and probably genetically derived

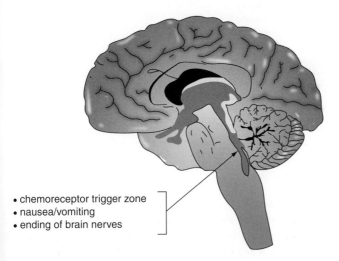

Figure 6.6. Sagittal view of the brain and anatomic localization of structures important for postoperative nausea and vomiting (PONV).

• chemoreceptor trigger zone
• nausea/vomiting
• ending of brain nerves

Table 6.2. Risk factors/causes for postoperative nausea and vomiting

Patient factors:	Female Individual, genetic Nonsmoker Motion sickness (more than average) and/or PONV by/previous general anesthesia Other: Low age, anxiety, dehydration
Surgical procedures with increased risk:	Intra-abdominal surgery (including laparoscopy, open gynecology) Middle ear surgery Strabismus surgery Tonsillectomy Surgery in face, neck (e.g., thyroid surgery) Long-lasting, invasive surgery with major cell destruction
Anesthesia and other drugs:	Inhalational anesthesia (isoflurane, sevoflurane, desflurane) Nitrous oxide Opioid effect postoperatively Neostigmine reversal of muscle relaxants

Simplified risk score (adapted from Apfel et al. [28]):

Risk factor	Score	Score sum
Female	1	Score=0: 10% risk
Nonsmoker	1	Score=1: 20% risk
History of PONV or travel sickness	1	Score=2: 40% risk
Postoperative opioid effect	1	Score=3: 60% risk
		Score=4: 80% risk

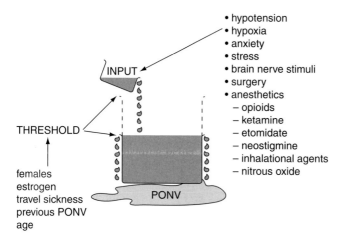

INPUT

THRESHOLD

females
estrogen
travel sickness
previous PONV
age

PONV

• hypotension
• hypoxia
• anxiety
• stress
• brain nerve stimuli
• surgery
• anesthetics
  – opioids
  – ketamine
  – etomidate
  – neostigmine
  – inhalational agents
  – nitrous oxide

Figure 6.7. Schematic model of PONV risk and threshold.

PONV is analogous to a bucket filled with water. When there is overflow, PONV will occur.

This risk of overflow (threshold) depends on the size of the bucket (i.e., the height of the bucket wall), which is smaller in females and patients with a genetic tendency for emesis, as evidenced by a history of previous PONV or strong travel sickness.

Whether the threshold is reached is determined by what is placed into the bucket, which are itemized in the list on the right.

differences in the threshold for PONV initiation are significant and in order to assess a patient's individual risk it is good practice to ask about their tendency to travel sickness and previous PONV. In children, it has been shown that a strong tendency to travel sickness or PONV in the parents is associated with a higher risk of postoperative vomiting in the child [7]. Emotional issues are also important, both conscious and subconscious memory and memory processing; anxiety, strong visual input, and recall of previous nausea (e.g., cytotoxic treatment) may evoke PONV symptoms.

Surgery always destroys cells, with the resultant outflow of potent proteins and cytokines into the bloodstream that reach the chemoreceptor-sensitive cells in the midbrain. Prolonged and/or extensive surgery and tissue destruction create a stronger input. Furthermore, surgery involving the gut and peritoneum (laparotomy, gynecologic surgery, laparoscopy) or other parts of the body innervated by brain nerves (ENT, eye, thyroid, neck, jaw, and face) will increase the risk of PONV. The use of a gastric tube after surgery may stimulate PONV, as may hypotension or hypoxia.

Drugs, food, and beverages may have a toxic and stimulating effect on the chemoreceptor zone when present in the blood, e.g., the emetic effects of cytotoxic cancer drugs, infected food, or alcohol. Potent inhalational agents (isoflurane, sevoflurane, desflurane, etc.) may have much the same effect. Nitrous oxide may also induce PONV, but the risk is not always evident in studies with an otherwise low baseline incidence. Reversal of neuromuscular block with neostigmine may provoke PONV, at least in doses of 40–50 µg/kg or more [8]. Use of propofol for maintenance of anesthesia or sedation seems to protect against PONV during the procedure and for some hours afterwards [9]. It seems that the protective effect of propofol relates to the plasma level, such that the higher the dose and the longer the drug is used, the longer the protective effect will last; ranging from 10–20 min after a single bolus to up to 2–5 h after prolonged use. There is also a blood level threshold for inducing PONV with opioids: residual opioids after anesthesia and opioid used to treat postoperative pain will increase the risk of PONV. Reduction or elimination of the opioid load by using loco-regional techniques for surgery will lower the PONV risk, as will the optimal use of nonopioid analgesics for postoperative analgesia (see Postoperative pain). It is disputed whether short-lasting opioids, such as remifentanil, induce an emetic effect for some time after they have been eliminated from the plasma, but data from sedation practice indicate that this is not the case [10].

For practical preoperative evaluation, the four Apfel–Koivuranta criteria for PONV risk may be very helpful [11] (Table 6.2), although the impact of surgery (invasiveness and duration) and the benefits of propofol use may be added.

For risk in children the simplified scoring of Eberhardt et al. may be useful [7]. This scoring system includes the length of surgery and strabismus surgery as risk factors, as well as parental PONV or emesis, although the aspect of propofol use versus inhalational agents is not addressed.

Nondrug treatment and prophylaxis of PONV

It has been shown that appropriate hydration will protect against PONV [12]. As even ambulatory patients for minor procedures are slightly dehydrated because of their preoperative fasting, it is good practice to always give about 500–1000 ml iv crystalloid to all patients, even for procedures that are short and have no anticipated blood loss. Hunger and thirst may cause PONV, thus it is wise not to extend the preoperative fasting period far beyond the standards of 2 h for fluid and 6 h for food. Some patients may become nauseated if they do not have their morning coffee or tea, and most of these patients will have ample time for their drink in the early morning without disobeying the 2 h fluid fasting rule. Postoperatively, many patients feel better after having drink or food, often within 30–60 min of an uneventful ambulatory case. The principle is to offer the patient the option of drinking or light food as

139

soon as they want it, rather than having strict rules about how much time should lapse before ingestion is allowed or required. There are reports of PONV occurring in patients who have been forced to drink or eat before they have felt like it, and it may be this that provoked the PONV [13].

Anxiety may sometimes cause PONV and may certainly exacerbate the distress caused by PONV from other reasons. Thus perioperative reassurance, distraction, and comforting may be of value in this context, as may occasionally an anxiolytic such as benzodiazepine.

Whether pain per se induces PONV is still disputed, but concomitant pain will certainly not make the feelings of nausea and overall wellbeing any better. Thus, routinely treating pain appropriately with nonopioid measures often reduces the reported discomfort from nausea. If an opioid is needed for pain treatment this should not be restricted; the approach is to give the opioid and observe. Sometimes the nausea will go away with the pain, even if opioid is given; but on other occasions the nausea will persist and then a specific anti-emetic drug should be given.

Hypoxia or hypotension may cause PONV, thus it is always good practice to check the pulse oximeter and measure the blood pressure when a patient complains of PONV.

A gastric tube will increase the risk of PONV in the awake patient. There are very few evidence-based indications for keeping a gastric tube in place after ambulatory surgery, thus usual practice is to limit the use of peroperative gastric tubes and routinely remove them before the patient emerges.

Strong movements may induce PONV, thus one should be gentle and careful when moving patients from the operating table, wheeling a bed or trolley, and also when mobilizing the patient to sitting or standing positions. Gentle handling, appropriate hydration, and perhaps ephedrine prophylaxis (see below) are good measures in this context, as is continuous verbal communication with the patient during movements.

In some patients causes of PONV that are not related to the procedure may be present, such as migraine, so a history of episodes of nausea in daily life is always useful to have to elucidate such causes.

Drug principles for prophylaxis and treatment of PONV [4,5]

Receptors that are stimulated by endogenous substances resulting in PONV have been identified in the chemoreceptor trigger zone: histamine, dopamine, serotonin, acetylcholine (muscarinic receptor), and opioid (Figure 6.8). Most anti-emetics are antagonists of these receptors. All these drugs work as both prophylaxis and treatment for the different types of nausea and vomiting (i.e., induced by toxins, movement, or emotions), but there are drug differences in terms of both effect profile and pharmacokinetic profile that mean their efficacy varies according to the patient and their particular circumstance. None of the present anti-emetics is fully effective; an effective response is usually seen in 20–50% of patients when given alone at the optimal dose. Thus, increasing the dose further will only increase the risk of side-effects; good practice is to use a multimodal approach by combining two to four different drug principles in high-risk patients when the one-drug treatment fails. By combining three to four drugs it is possible to relieve the symptoms in nearly all patients. By careful planning of surgery, anesthetic method, nonopioid pain treatment, and appropriate PONV prophylaxis the risk should approach less than 5–10% in modern ambulatory anesthesia. Prophylaxis may be achieved by both oral and iv administration, however the oral route is

Table 6.3. Drug principles for anti-emetic therapy

Drug	Onset	Duration	Effect	
			Prophylaxis	Treatment
Metoclopramide	++	+ (3–6 h)	+ (short lasting)	++
Neuroleptics	++	+++ (12–24 h)	+++	+++
5HT3 (serotonin) antagonists	++	++++ (18–24 h)	+++	+++
Glucocorticoid	–(h)	++++	+++	(+) slow
Ephedrine	++(+)	+ (1–3 h)	++ (sc or im)	++
Antihistamine	+	++(+)	++	++
Anticholinergics (scopolamine)	+	+++	++	+

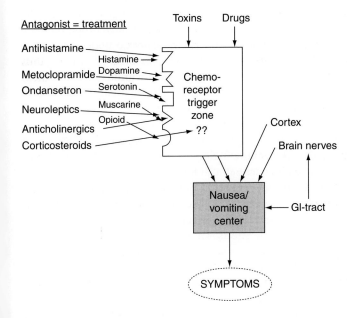

Figure 6.8. Schematic drawing of receptors important for stimulation of the chemoreceptor trigger zone.

not very appropriate for treatment. Nevertheless, if the patient can keep a sublingual tablet this may be an option, as with ondansetron. Although suppositories have a very unpredictable rate and amount of absorption, this may be the only route available with overt PONV after discharge and removal of the iv line.

Notes on relevant anti-emetic drugs [4], Table 6.3

Metoclopramide

This is a dopamine receptor antagonist that is also a serotonin antagonist at doses that are 4–5 times higher than those used normally. Standard treatment in adults with PONV is 10–20 mg iv, which may be repeated 3–4 times per day.

Similar dosing may also be used orally (tablet, mixture) or rectally. The effect of a single dose is fairly short-lived, at best up to 6–10 h [14]. For that reason the drug is not that good for prophylaxis, but has documented effects for 3–6 h after a minimum dose of 20 mg. Side-effects at these doses are quite minor and rare, but include extrapyramidal movements, dysphoria, and restlessness.

Neuroleptics

These are also dopamine antagonists and some of them have antihistaminergic and anti-cholinergic effects as well. The problem with many neuroleptics is a sedative hypnotic dose-dependent effect, which is something you want to avoid in the early postoperative phase. The focus has thus been on low-dose haloperidol (1.0–2.5 mg iv) [15] and especially droperidol, which has efficacy without measurable sedation at doses of 0.67–1.25 mg in adults. The effect is long-lasting, up to 24 h, thus the drug is much used for prophylaxis. Side-effects are rare, but include extrapyramidal movements. Disturbed night sleep and dysphoria after a single dose have been described, and some claim that haloperidol is a better alternative in this respect for treatment in the postoperative period. Much debate, especially in the USA, took place after a few reports of dysrhythmia after droperidol and prolonged Q-T intervals in the ECG with low-dose droperidol. Dedicated studies are unable to confirm these initial reports and so droperidol should now be declared safe with regards to cardiac dysrhythmia [16], and an ECG is not required prior to droperidol administration. Other neuroleptics can be used instead, for instance dixyrazine (10 mg orally), prochlorper-azine, or perphenazine.

Serotonin antagonists

A new class of drugs specially designed as anti-emetics has arisen in the form of type 3 serotonin receptor (5HT3) antagonists. They are efficient against PONV and emesis asso-ciated with chemotherapy, but are not very effective against motion sickness. Compared with neuroleptics they seem to be more effective against vomiting, whereas the overall anti-emetic effect is comparable with that provided by neuroleptics or corticosteroids. Apart from minor headache or stomach spasm, they have few side-effects. The cost is still high for some of these drugs, but ondansetron has recently become generic and cheap, and the same is likely to happen shortly with the others. Conventional 5HT3 antagonists are effective for both prophylaxis and treatment for about 24 h, whereas ongoing pharmaceutical development may result in drugs with an even more prolonged action. Ondansetron (4 mg iv for prophylaxis and 1–2 mg for treatment) is the one that has been used the most and is the best documented, but the characteristics of granisetron, dolasetron, and tropisetron seem to be very similar to those of ondansetron.

Glucocorticoids

These drugs have been around for quite some time, but recognition of their anti-emetic effect in small doses with the benefit of barely any side-effects has taken 10–20 years to emerge. However, the mechanism of their anti-emetic effect remains under dispute and unclear. The onset of effect is slow, emerging over a period of hours, and these drugs are best for prophylaxis when given early after anesthetic induction. The most documented effect is with dexamethasone, 3–4 mg iv [17], but betamethasone or methylprednisolone also work well in comparable doses [18]. By doubling or tripling the dose, corticosteroids are also good analgesics (see Postoperative pain). A feature characteristic of most dexamethasone preparations is strong genital or perineal burning aching, which is quite frequently observed when given by fast iv to an awake patient.

Ephedrine

The mechanism of ephedrine's anti-emetic effect is also under dispute. Ephedrine may prevent the hypotension and emesis precipitated by movement and mobilization, but studies also show that it has a true anti-emetic effect in normotensive patients where no movement is involved. By intravenous dosing of 5–10 mg (adults) the effect is short lasting (15–30 min) but without significant tachycardia. A more prolonged effect from 0.5 mg/kg subcutaneously may last up to 3 h [19].

Antihistamines

In this drug class, the traditional antihistamines that penetrate the blood–brain barrier and have a sedative side-effect profile are the most efficacious for anti-emesis: promethazine, hydroxyzine, or cyclizine. While antihistamines are much used for travel sickness and motion sickness, they are used less in the perioperative setting, partly because their side-effects of a dry mouth and sedation are not desirable in the postoperative phase. They may still be a valuable option for PONV treatment when other principles of drug action have already been exploited [20].

Anticholinergics

As described for antihistamines above, the anticholinergics that have a centrally acting sedative effect are also anti-emetic. Scopolamine [21], as either a skin pad or injection, is effective but will cause a dry mouth and significant sedation in most patients. In some places scopolamine is combined with morphine for sedation or premedication, but even with scopolamine some patients are nauseated by the morphine [22,23].

NK1 inhibitors

The NK1 receptor antagonists form a new class of anti-emetic drugs, which have proven to be very effective against cytostatic-induced emesis and are being used increasingly for PONV [24,25]. They seem to be equally effective as the 5HT3 antagonists in terms of strength and duration for nausea, and are potentially better for vomiting [24]. While they are still expensive, they may be used as an alternative for both prophylaxis and treatment in cases where the conventional multimodal approach fails.

Miscellaneous

Acupressure and *electrostimulation* have been demonstrated to have significant anti-emetic effects linked to their application to traditional acupuncture stimulus sites [26].

While reversal of opioid-induced PONV may be facilitated by *naloxone* the strategy is not usually deemed successful as the patient's pain also returns. However, some preliminary reports have also suggested a potential anti-emetic property of the peripherally acting opioid antagonist *methylnaltrexone* [27], which does not have an impact on centrally mediated pain relief.

Practical approach

Prophylaxis

Two alternative approaches may be used: (1) to establish fixed prophylaxis for all patients with certain procedures or (2) to make individual evaluations of each patient and case based on their specific risk factors. If the risk is considered to be in the range of 20–40% single-drug prophylaxis may do; in the range 30–60%, use double-drug prophylaxis; above 50%, adopt a triple-drug prophylactic approach. Typically we use dexamethasone as single-drug prophylaxis if not contraindicated (some orthopedic procedures), alternatively use ondansetron. These drugs are combined for double-drug prophylaxis; if one is contraindicated, replace it with droperidol. For triple-drug prophylaxis all three are combined. In high-risk patients, but also otherwise when feasible, focus is on propofol-based general anesthesia, optimal loco-regional techniques, avoidance of nitrous oxide and inhalational agents, as well as optimal nonopioid pain prophylaxis and treatment. The prophylactic drugs are most efficient when given at the end of the procedure; the exception is glucocorticoid, which should be given shortly after induction of anesthesia in order to be effective at emergence. We also use to give droperidol before the start of the procedure, not only to avoid a potential sedative effect during emergence but also to have good ECG monitoring for any potential Q-T problems during the case (see above); mostly for medicolegal reasons as the existence of such problems is highly disputable.

Treatment

Good practice is to first correct for any dehydration, hypotension, hypoxia, gastric tube, pain, and anxiety if any of these are present. Then one should assess which prophylactic drug(s) the patient has received. Treatment should then start with drugs other than those used for prophylaxis, which, it should be assumed, are still working. Our routine is to start with metoclopramide 10–20 mg, wait for 5–10 min and then proceed with ondansetron if this is not still active in the patient, or use haloperidol or another neuroleptic. Ephedrine may also be tried, especially if the emetic episode is triggered by movement, hypotension, or mobilization. A glucocorticoid (dexamethasone) may also be useful for long-term treatment, but should not be expected to have an effect initially.

If the droperidol + glucocorticoid + neuroleptic options have been used for prophylaxis, then treatment with metoclopramide, ephedrine, and promethazine may be viable options.

References

1. Imasogie N, Chung F. Risk factors for prolonged stay after ambulatory surgery: economic considerations. *Curr Opin Anaesthesiol* 2002;**15**:245–9.

2. Skledar SJ, Williams BA, Vallejo MC, et al. Eliminating postoperative nausea and vomiting in outpatient surgery with multimodal strategies including low doses of nonsedating, off-patent antiemetics: is "zero tolerance" achievable? *Sci World J* 2007;**7**:959–77.

3. Watcha MF, White PF. Postoperative nausea and vomiting. Its etiology, treatment, and prevention. *Anesthesiology* 1992;**77**:162–84.

4. Gan TJ, Meyer TA, Apfel CC, et al. Society for Ambulatory Anesthesia guidelines for the management of postoperative nausea and vomiting. *Anesth Analg* 2007;**105**:1615–28, table.

5. Bustos F, Semeraro C, Lopez S, Giner M. Management of post-operative nausea and vomiting in ambulatory surgery. In: Lemos P, Jarrett P, Philip B, eds. *Day Surgery – Development and Practice*, London: IAAS, 2006: 229–40.

6. Raeder J. [Postoperative nausea and vomiting.] *Tidsskr Nor Laegeforen* 2005;**125**:1831–2.

7. Eberhart LH, Geldner G, Kranke P, et al. The development and validation of a risk score to predict the probability of postoperative vomiting in pediatric patients. *Anesth Analg* 2004;**99**:1630–7, table.

8. Lovstad RZ, Thagaard KS, Berner NS, Raeder JC. Neostigmine 50 µg kg^{-1} with glycopyrrolate increases postoperative nausea in women after laparoscopic gynaecological

surgery. *Acta Anaesthesiol Scand* 2001;**45**:495–500.

9. Gauger PG, Shanks A, Morris M, et al. Propofol decreases early postoperative nausea and vomiting in patients undergoing thyroid and parathyroid operations. *World J Surg* 2008;**32**:1525–34.

10. Servin FS, Raeder JC, Merle JC, et al. Remifentanil sedation compared with propofol during regional anaesthesia. *Acta Anaesthesiol Scand* 2002;**46**:309–15.

11. Apfel CC, Kranke P, Eberhart LH, et al. Comparison of predictive models for postoperative nausea and vomiting. *Br J Anaesth* 2002;**88**:234–40.

12. Maharaj CH, Kallam SR, Malik A, et al. Preoperative intravenous fluid therapy decreases postoperative nausea and pain in high risk patients. *Anesth Analg* 2005;**100**:675–82, table.

13. Charoenkwan K, Phillipson G, Vutyavanich T. Early versus delayed oral fluids and food for reducing complications after major abdominal gynecologic surgery. *Cochrane Database Syst Rev* 2007;CD004508.

14. Quaynor H, Raeder JC. Incidence and severity of postoperative nausea and vomiting are similar after metoclopramide 20 mg and ondansetron 8 mg given by the end of laparoscopic cholecystectomies. *Acta Anaesthesiol Scand* 2002;**46**:109–13.

15. Wang TF, Liu YH, Chu CC, et al. Low-dose haloperidol prevents post-operative nausea and vomiting after ambulatory laparoscopic surgery. *Acta Anaesthesiol Scand* 2008;**52**:280–4.

16. White PF, Abrao J. Drug-induced prolongation of the QT interval: what's the point? *Anesthesiology* 2006;**104**:386–7.

17. Henzi I, Walder B, Tramer MR. Dexamethasone for the prevention of postoperative nausea and vomiting: a quantitative systematic review. *Anesth Analg* 2000;**90**:186–94.

18. Aasboe V, Raeder JC, Groegaard B. Betamethasone reduces postoperative pain and nausea after ambulatory surgery. *Anesth Analg* 1998;**87**:319–23.

19. Hagemann E, Halvorsen A, Holgersen O, et al. Intramuscular ephedrine reduces emesis during the first three hours after abdominal hysterectomy. *Acta Anaesthesiol Scand* 2000;**44**:107–11.

20. Habib AS, Gan TJ. The effectiveness of rescue antiemetics after failure of prophylaxis with ondansetron or droperidol: a preliminary report. *J Clin Anesth* 2005;**17**:62–5.

21. White PF, Tang J, Song D, et al. Transdermal scopolamine: an alternative to ondansetron and droperidol for the prevention of postoperative and postdischarge emetic symptoms. *Anesth Analg* 2007;**104**:92–6.

22. Raeder JC, Breivik H. Premedication with midazolam in out-patient general anaesthesia. A comparison with morphine-scopolamine and placebo. *Acta Anaesthesiol Scand* 1987;**31**:509–14.

23. Kranke P, Morin AM, Roewer N, et al. The efficacy and safety of transdermal scopolamine for the prevention of postoperative nausea and vomiting: a quantitative systematic review. *Anesth Analg* 2002;**95**:133–43, table.

24. Diemunsch P, Joshi GP, Brichant JF. Neurokinin-1 receptor antagonists in the prevention of postoperative nausea and vomiting. *Br J Anaesth* 2009;**103**:7–13.

25. Gan TJ, Apfel CC, Kovac A, et al. A randomized, double-blind comparison of the NK1 antagonist, aprepitant, versus ondansetron for the prevention of postoperative nausea and vomiting. *Anesth Analg* 2007;**104**:1082–9, tables.

26. White PF, Hamza MA, Recart A, et al. Optimal timing of acustimulation for antiemetic prophylaxis as an adjunct to ondansetron in patients undergoing plastic surgery. *Anesth Analg* 2005;**100**:367–72.

27. Moss J, Rosow CE. Development of peripheral opioid antagonists; new insights into opioid effects. *Mayo Clin Proc* 2008;**83**:1116–30.

28. Apfel CC, Laara E, Koivuranta M, et al. A simplified risk score for predicting postoperative nausea and vomiting: conclusions from cross-validations between two centers. *Anesthesiology* 1999;**91**:693–700.

Other postoperative problems [1]
Shivering

Shivering may occur because of hypothermia, with core temperatures below 35–36°. Even after short ambulatory surgery many patients will feel cold after emergence. They have been lying still without muscular activity on an operating table, often not that well covered with blankets. Furthermore, general anesthesia and also neuraxial blocks (epidural, spinal) will cause a shift in body heat from the core to the surface and this may induce shivering in spite of draping and a warm temperature in the room [2]. Shivering during normothermia may also be the result of anesthetic drug influence. A high incidence is described after inhalational anesthesia, worst with isoflurane. Shivering may also occur after propofol-based anesthesia, but less than after potent inhalational drugs. Shivering will increase the oxygen consumption and will be unpleasant for the patient, also because movements in the surgical wound usually occur. Whereas most opioids reduce shivering [3], iv pethidine (meperidine) seems to have a specific and higher efficacy in doses of 10–20 mg iv in the adult [4]. If meperidine does not work (10 mg given twice) the next option is to use clonidine 150 μg iv.

Pruritus

Dry skin, washing, draping, and also generalized allergic reactions may cause postoperative pruritus, which may be treated causally by local skin treatment (hydrocortisone emulsion) or iv antihistamines (e.g., promethazine 12.5 mg iv). Systemic opioids and especially epidural or spinal opioid may also cause pruritus. While a very carefully titrated and low-dose injection of naloxone 0.05–0.1 mg may be efficient against opioid-induced pruritus, this option should always be evaluated against the risk of elucidating pain. Some reports of success with a peripherally acting opioid antagonist, such as methylnaltrexone [5], have occurred recently; if efficient, this will not be at the cost of renewed pain.

With mild symptoms, it may be wise to wait and see before giving specific drugs, as the condition is self-limiting.

Urinary retention

Urinary retention may occur in any patient after surgery and anesthesia, but is more frequent in elderly men and in patients having surgical procedures in the lower abdomen and perineal areas. While 500–1000 ml of basic iv fluid replacement is a good rule for all ambulatory patients (due to its anti-emetic effect), care should be taken not to give more fluid than necessary peroperatively. Also, patients should always empty their bladder before their surgical procedure and before being taken to the operating theater. Usually there is no indication for a bladder catheter peroperatively in ambulatory patients, but this should be considered individually for procedures of more than 5–6 h planned duration. With some gynecologic procedures a catheter may be a surgical requirement.

When there is no micturition postoperatively it is wise to establish by scan whether the patient has a full bladder before proceeding to catheterization. If the bladder is not filled, catheterization should wait; many patients will have a lowered urinary production for many hours after a surgical procedure and may not void until late in the evening. However, for those patients suspected of having urinary retention due to neuraxial opioid or (rarely) systemic opioids, the bladder should be checked for overdistension and, if in doubt, a catheter should be inserted. An alternative may be to try naloxone or methylnaltrexone (see above).

Many units do not require the patient to void before discharge, as long as they have not had a neuraxial block or are otherwise at high risk of urinary retention. Nevertheless, when a patient is discharged to home without first having voided it is very important to inform the patient and chaperone to contact health personnel if voiding does not occur in the first 6–8 h after surgery.

Somnolescence

Usually this is caused by the residual effects of anesthetic drugs and should not warrant any specific actions apart from checking the dosing reports, providing good monitoring of vital functions, and stimulating the patient if necessary. It is usually well worth spending 10–20 min at the bedside applying the jaw thrust and perhaps moving to careful bag-and-mask assistance before proceeding to re-intubation or reinsertion of the LMA and ventilator treatment. In selected cases opioid antagonists (i.e., naloxone) or benzodiazepine (i.e., flumazenil) may be tried; dosing with careful titration of 0.1 mg iv at a time may be appropriate for both. If a patient has a significant emergence on one of these antagonists, one should keep in mind that there may be a reccurrence of sedation after 30–60 min as the effects of the antagonists are usually more short-lasting than those of the parent drug.

Postoperative agitation

Postoperative agitation or delirium may occur in any patient after general anesthesia, but occurs more frequently in the elderly or in patients with an alcohol, drug, or narcotic abuse problem. Such problems may not always be on the chart as some of these patients are reluctant to report them. Regular alcohol abuse in particular may emerge as an unexpected postoperative agitation problem in otherwise healthy and normally functioning patients. When agitation is induced by drug or narcotic withdrawal, a good combined diagnostic and therapeutic approach is to titrate carefully either a benzodiazepine (diazepam 2–3 mg iv) or fentanyl (0.05 mg iv). If the reaction continues or there is a suspicion of alcohol withdrawal, titrated doses of haloperidol 1–2 mg iv at a time may be attempted. In cases of severe and overt alcohol abstinence, clonidine may also be tried, 2–4 µg/kg iv for titration. Haloperidol may also be tried for agitative delirium without any known causes.

Postoperative anxiety

This condition should always be sought in patients with continuous shivering, crying, or inappropriate effect of ordinary pain treatment. Good nursing care is a key issue; try to calm down and reassure the patient and try to gather whether there is a problem with pain or another specific problem calling for specific therapy. If the above are ruled out or if doubt remains, and reassuring care does not help, a test dose of diazepam 2–4 mg iv is often a good way to continue before re-evaluating the patient.

General postoperative care

Postoperative care is often divided into four phases:

1. Immediate care in the postanesthesia care unit (PACU)
2. Further hospital care in the phase II recovery or step-down unit
3. Discharge
4. Postdischarge care.

Immediate care in the postanesthesia care (PACU) unit

In the ambulatory care setting, patients almost always arrive in the PACU with a free airway, breathing spontaneously, and with stable hemodynamics, but occasionally initial support of these vital functions is required. Sometimes patients may be fully alert, awake, and already fulfilling the PACU discharge criteria (see below) and for that reason go directly to the phase II or step-down unit. This so-called fast tracking may be an important economic issue in those hospitals that have separate billing for PACU services, as otherwise these patients may go to the PACU regardless of need and stay there for a short time even though technical monitoring is not required.

The routine setup in the PACU is to have the patient initially flat, lying on their side (if surgery permits) in a bed or on a trolley, and to have a continuous ECG, pulse oximetry, and regular noninvasive BP readings, with documentation of values every 10 min as long as the patient is unconscious. Usually oxygen supplement should also be given as long as the patient is unconscious, and sometimes for longer if the readings are hard to keep above the 90–92% level without. In stable children and in awake adults the monitoring may be reduced to pulse oximetry unless there are special indications for blood pressure or ECG.

The nursing care will otherwise include a very low speed infusion of crystalloid, wound checks, draping and perhaps drains, as well as monitoring and iv treatment of pain or PONV. As the patient wakes up there should be attempts to wean them off oxygen, to sip water, and to half sit up in bed with their head elevated. Furthermore, patients should be regularly assessed to see whether they are ready for PACU discharge (Table 6.4). Once ready, the patient may either be physically discharged or remain in the PACU, but without monitoring and otherwise encouraged to mobilize and drink/eat as in the phase II recovery.

In general all criteria should be fulfilled, but exceptions may be warranted based on the patient's preoperative condition or other special circumstances, evaluated for each case separately.

Further hospital care in the phase II recovery or step-down unit

In this unit the patient should be able to sit or reside in a resting chair. No technical monitoring or iv infusion should be necessary, but the patient should not be left alone in the room without an adult, a responsible person, present. In this phase the patient should be offered a drink and a light meal; furthermore, preparations should be made for discharge in terms of information exchange and logistics. Usually it is wise to keep the iv cannula in place until the patient is ready for discharge. Equipment and drugs for monitoring and support of

Table 6.4. Scoring system to determine whether the patient can be discharged from the PACU or bypass the PACU (if criteria are fulfilled before arriving there). Modified from White and Song [6]

1. Awake and oriented, or easily arousable and able to rest further in a chair

2. Able to sit and to move all extremities

3. Blood pressure and heart rate stable and with acceptable values (i.e., no clinical signs of hypotension or bradycardia, no new development of hypertension or arrhythmia)

4. Breathing stable; able to breathe deeply and able to cough

5. Oxygen saturation of at least 90% on room air

6. No or mild pain or nausea, no vomiting

vital functions as well as analgesics and anti-emetics should be readily available if needed. Exceptions may be made for small children and psychiatric patients, who may be very distressed by the iv cannula, which then may be removed once they are discharged from the PACU.

When a patient fulfills the discharge criteria (Table 6.5), he or she may be discharged. In general all criteria should be fulfilled, but exceptions may be warranted based on the patient's preoperative condition or other special circumstances, evaluated individually.

Discharge

Before the discharge (Table 6.5) can be fulfilled, the patient should be free of their iv cannula and dressed in their own clothes. The patient and chaperone should have both oral and written information about the following:

1. Surgery, included in a written report to be kept by them in case they need to contact health personnel.
2. Anesthesia, any special events (sore throat, muscle ache), and general precautions: not driving until the next day, not taking important decisions or signing documents, not drinking alcohol.
3. Advice on appropriate daily activities, rehabilitation, training, and precautions.
4. Information about wound care, change of dressings, when showers can be taken, etc.
5. Information about common side-effects and concerns: some stained blood in the dressing, type of expected pain (e.g., in the shoulder after a laparoscopy), minor fever during the first 24–48 h.
6. Information about unexpected symptoms that should prompt the patient to contact health personnel: fresh bleeding from a wound, fainting, increasing fever after day 2,

Table 6.5. Checklist to determine whether the outpatient can be discharged from hospital to home or a hospital-hotel. Modified from Chung [7]

1. Vital signs (breathing, blood pressure, heart rate) must be stable and consistent with the patient's preoperative condition
2. Patient must be able to ambulate at a preoperative level (excluding special measures due to surgery or dressing) and be able to sit in a car for the anticipated time of home travel. Motor block after spinal or epidural anesthesia must be fully resolved
3. The level of pain or nausea should be minimal, acceptable to the patient, and lend itself to further control by oral (or perhaps rectal) medication
4. The patient should have no ongoing bleeding and no other unforeseen surgical problems which may be incompatible with a safe postdischarge course
5. The patient should accept to be discharged
6. The patient should have an adult escort with him/her on the way home[a] and at home until the next day
7. The patient should not be expected to have any problems drinking and voiding. The best test is of course that the patient drinks and voids before leaving, but they should not be forced to do so, unless there is a special indication (see discussion of voiding in text). If a patient is discharged without drinking and voiding, they should have thorough instruction on how to behave and of the signs of potential concern after discharge.

[a] The escort may be a responsible taxi driver.

increasing size of or pain in the abdomen, problems with drinking/eating/voiding, strong pain, continued vomiting.

7. Clear instructions on where to call (the surgeon, the unit, the hospital, other health personnel) for 24 h service in case of problems and questions.

8. Instructions on how to deal with pain prophylaxis and extra medication for pain or PONV. The instructions should be accompanied by any tablets the patient may need until at least the next day, when someone can go to the pharmacy (also provide prescriptions for extra analgesics needed after day 2). Alternatively, it can be arranged for the patient to buy these drugs before surgery.

9. Declaration of necessary sick leave for authorities and employer.

10. Appointment for an outpatient follow-up consultation, when this is regarded as appropriate: for medical reasons, for perceived patient quality and reassurance, or for quality assurance.

Postdischarge care

Postoperative care may be anything from no measures beyond appropriate on-call availability 24 h a day, through telephones, questionnaires, to outpatient consultation.

On-call availability

It is absolutely essential for the safety and success of ambulatory practice to have a well-defined and clear setup for where the patient or relatives can call in case of questions or problems 24 h a day. As the ambulatory unit by definition is closed for part of the day, an alternative location must provide a readily accessible, friendly, and up-to-date telephone service. For office-based practice, small units and special cases, this may be the surgeon's cell phone, but this may be demanding for the surgeon and sometimes also unreliable as cell phones and signal coverage may fail. A better system is for the service to be provided at a nearby emergency unit with full access to patient data and surgical reports.

Phone call from the unit or the hospital the day after

Many units make routine calls to all ambulatory patients the day after surgery, whereas others only do so for selected cases. The idea is to ensure that all questions and instructions are followed, to hear about any problems or questions, and also to obtain data for quality assurance. If a call is planned, it may be wise to tell the patient about the calling routine, not only to allow them the chance to prepare their own questions but also to avoid any anxiety prompted by an unexpected call from the hospital. The call may be made by a nurse, the surgeon, or the anesthesiologist. It may be sensible to have a structured setup for questions and also to have the option for the patient to come forward with spontaneous input. With a "next-day" call most immediate problems will be dealt with nicely, but such a call will not be informative about the occurrence of infection or thrombosis, which usually happen on day 3 or later; therefore, their usefulness is limited when evaluating outcome. If the patient does not answer, it may be possible to leave a message on an answer phone, to talk with a relative instead, or one might assume that their not answering means that they are not interested.

Some items which may be included in the interview are listed below:

a. Any problems (pain, nausea?) during home travel?

b. Extent of pain, use of analgesics and satisfaction with regime?

c. Any nausea or vomiting?

d. Any problems with the wound and dressings?

e. Problems with eating, drinking, natural functions?

f. Degree of mobilization?

g. Quality and amount of night sleep, daytime sleep, or sedation?

h. Need for contact with health care professionals?

Written questionnaire for the patient

This is more a tool for quality assurance for the unit, as the patient will not get rapid feedback on worrisome answers for many days. Nevertheless, a questionnaire may be very useful for this purpose as it is more standardized than an interview and will be less time-consuming for the personnel at the ambulatory unit. The questionnaire may be sent with the patient or sent to them afterwards. It may be for next-day completion, or for completion after 1–2 weeks or even after 1–3 months, in order to obtain more outcome data. To be successful the questionnaire should not be too cumbersome (yes/no answers, or ticking alternatives) and it should be accompanied by a prestamped envelope addressed to the unit. Lack of patient response can cause problems and may be handled by sending a gentle reminder, and motivating the patient to answer before leaving the unit.

Outpatient consultation

As this is time-consuming for both doctor and patient there should be a health indication for such a consultation, although it may also be part of a more dedicated quality assurance project or a research project. The benefit with a visit is that much more information can be obtained, because some types of information are difficult to gather by mail or phone, such as wound healing, absence of infection, standardized degree of rehabilitation, etc.

References

1. Awad I, Chung F. Post-operative recovery and discharge. In: Lemos P, Jarrett P, Philip B, eds. *Day Surgery – Development and Practice*, London: IAAS, 2006: 241–56.

2. Sessler DI. Temperature monitoring and perioperative thermoregulation. *Anesthesiology* 2008;**109**:318–38.

3. Alfonsi P, Hongnat JM, Lebrault C, Chauvin M. The effects of pethidine, fentanyl and lignocaine on postanaesthetic shivering. *Anaesthesia* 1995;**50**:214–17.

4. Kranke P, Eberhart LH, Roewer N, Tramer MR. Pharmacological treatment of postoperative shivering: a quantitative systematic review of randomized controlled trials. *Anesth Analg* 2002;**94**:453–60, table.

5. Moss J, Rosow CE. Development of peripheral opioid antagonists' new insights into opioid effects. *Mayo Clin Proc* 2008;**83**:1116–30.

6. White PF, Song D. New criteria for fast-tracking after outpatient anesthesia: a comparison with the modified Aldrete's scoring system. *Anesth Analg* 1999;**88**:1069–72.

7. Chung F. Recovery pattern and home-readiness after ambulatory surgery. *Anesth Analg* 1995;**80**:896–902.

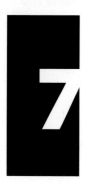

7 Practical recipes, from start (pre-op) to end (discharge)

The "recipes" in this chapter are based on discussions of issues in previous chapters. In anesthesia there are certainly many different ways of achieving good results, but we have to choose among them in our everyday practice.

These are some of my choices in my setting. Unless otherwise stated, assume the case is an adult patient with no special issues to consider.

Standard total intravenous anesthesia and target control infusion (TCI) for procedures of 15 min to 5 h

This is my standard method for adults in a setting with target control infusion (TCI) pumps for remifentanil and propofol, and no inhalational agent. TCI remifentanil follows the Minto effect-site model; TCI propofol, the Marsh effect-site model (modified short $T_{1/2}$ k_{eO} – the time taken for 50% equilibration from plasma to effect site – of Struys). Pumps are programmed with ideal weight, height – 100 (cm) for males or height – 105 (cm) for females. The infusion setup with valves is shown in Figure 7.1. Using this setup, the pumps, syringes, and lines can be used for one full working day for all patients, changing just the valves and infusion lines for each new patient. It has been shown that retrograde contamination may occur through a one-valve system, but with a double-valve system and unidirectional flow such contamination is not described.

In the obese I use the corrected ideal weight (= ideal weight + 20% of difference between real and ideal weight).

Premedication

a. **Anxiolysis**: usually none. If the patient is very anxious I give midazolam tablets 7.5 mg orally 1–2 h beforehand, or diazepam 5–10 mg orally if more than 2 h ahead. If surgery is scheduled in less than 1 h, I consider (only for the very anxious) inserting an iv line when the patient is in the holding area and giving 1–2 mg midazolam iv and asking a nurse to monitor.

b. **Analgesic prophylaxis**: paracetamol + nonsteroidal anti-inflammatory drug (NSAID) or cyclooxygenase II (COX-II) inhibitor as a routine:
   If more than 1 h to start of anesthesia:
   - Paracetamol tablets:
     2 g if > 60 kg weight and < 60 years
     1.5 g if > 60 years or < 60 kg weight
   - Diclofenac 100 mg if not contraindicated (75 mg if < 60 kg weight or > 60 years)
   - Celecoxib 200 mg is given instead of diclofenac if there is concern about potential peroperative bleeding or hematoma (plastic surgery, breast surgery) or relative

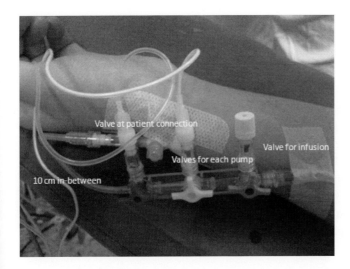

Figure 7.1. Unidirectional valves will ensure that no drugs, blood from the patient, or contamination will diffuse retrogradely. The lines from the pumps will be used for the next patient, but all valves, other lines, and infusion bags will be changed.

contraindications to traditional NSAIDs are present, such as previous gastrointestinal ulcer or strong allergy.

If less than 1 h to start of surgery is planned:
- No oral analgesics but give similar drugs iv after the start of anesthesia instead (see below, paragraph (d) under induction)

Induction

a. Use one iv line (dorsum of hand or crook of elbow to avoid ache from propofol), start to run in Ringer's crystalloid solution from a 1000 ml bag for induction, one-way valves and three-way couplings (see Figure 7.1). Start with propofol TCI of 1–1.5 μg/ml for sedation as soon as is feasible.

   Put on ECG, BP cuff, pulse oximeter, and note baseline values.

b. **Induction**: propofol target of 4.5 μg/ml, then immediately start remifentanil to target 6 ng/ml if laryngeal mask airway (LMA) is planned, or 8 ng/ml if endotracheal tube is planned. (If the patient is > 60 years I reduce the remifentanil target by 10–50%.) Ask the patient to breathe oxygen deeply by mask; assist as needed.

   After 2–3 min the patient's jaw feels relaxed and the LMA or tracheal tube may be inserted (a rule of thumb is for a total dose of about 1.5–2 mg/kg propofol, and remifentanil 1.5–2.5 μg/kg for LMA or 3–4 μg/kg for endotracheal tube).

c. Put in LMA or endotracheal tube.

d. Turn propofol down to 2.2 μg/ml and remifentanil to 4 ng/ml while waiting for surgery to start. Give dexamethasone 8 mg and droperidol 1.25 mg iv (droperidol may be skipped if the risk of postoperative nausea and vomiting (PONV) is low, or if the Apfel score is 1 or 0).

   If the patient did not receive paracetamol or NSAID/COX-II inhibitor tablets for premedication, give paracetamol 1 g as an iv infusion. If there is no risk of bleeding, give ketorolac 30 mg as the NSAID; if there is a risk of bleeding (or conventional NSAID is inferior in other aspects) I either give parecoxib 40 mg or wait until hemostasis is ensured before giving ketorolac.

e. At 30–60 s before the start of surgery, increase remifentanil to 6–12 ng/ml, depending upon both the anticipated level of surgical stress and the patient's reaction (blood pressure (BP) drop, heart rate) during induction.

Maintenance

a. Keep propofol in the 1.8–2.2 μg/ml range as a baseline drug for sleep. Do not let it fall below 1.8 μg/ml, otherwise sudden emergence may occur. Raise the propofol to 2.5–3.0 μg/ml at the start if the patient opens their eyes or moves despite a low BP, low heart rate, and adequate remifentanil level.

b. Remifentanil should be adjusted freely according to the patient's sensitivity and strength of surgical stimulation; anything from 4 to 15 (or even 20) ng/ml as needed.

c. Ventilation by volume control, tidal volume, 0.5–0.7 ml/kg ideal weight, frequency 12–16 breaths/min, peak end-expiratory pressure (PEEP) 4 cmH$_2$O, and fractional inspired oxygen (FiO_2) 40%.

End of case

a. Ensure the surgeon infiltrates all relevant wound structures with bupivacaine 2.5 mg/ml, 15–20 ml as needed. If more than 20 ml is needed, ropivacaine 2 mg/ml should be used instead (lower toxicity). Be generous with local anesthesia.

b. Give ondansetron 4 mg if the PONV risk is considered medium or high.

c. Give fentanyl 50–100 μg iv (to ensure against immediate pain as remifentanil is very rapidly eliminated).

d. Turn the TCI of propofol and remifentanil to zero.

e. Be ready to take over ventilation and to remove the LMA or tube as soon as the patient responds.

f. Ask patient if they have any pain; if positive, give another dose of fentanyl 50 μg.

Alternative to 7.1: TIVA, with TCI + nitrous oxide

This alternative is similar to recipe 7.1, with the exception of the following paragraphs:

Induction

d. Start nitrous oxide; 4 l/min in 2 l/min oxygen; after 10 min turn down nitrous oxide to 2 l/min and oxygen to 1 l/min if you have a circulating ventilator system with a scavenger. Otherwise, maintain levels at 4+2 l/min.

Turn propofol down to 1.8 μg/ml and remifentanil to 4 ng/ml while waiting for surgery to start. Give dexamethasone 8 mg and droperidol 1.25 mg iv (droperidol may be skipped if the PONV risk is low, or the Apfel score is 1 or 0).

If the patient did not receive paracetamol or NSAID/COX-II inhibitor tablets for premedication, then paracetamol 1 g is given as an iv infusion. If there is no risk of bleeding, give ketorolac 30 mg as the NSAID; if there is a risk of bleeding (or conventional NSAID is inferior in other aspects), I either give parecoxib 40 mg or I wait until hemostasis is ensured before giving ketorolac.

Maintenance

a. Keep propofol in the 1.5–2.0 µg/ml range as a baseline drug for sleep. Do not let it fall below 1.5 µg/ml, otherwise sudden emergence may occur. Raise the propofol to 2.5 µg/ml at the start if the patient opens their eyes or moves despite a low BP, low heart rate, and adequate remifentanil level.

End of case

c. Turn the TCI of propofol and remifentanil to zero.
Turn nitrous oxide to 0, and give oxygen 6 l/min for at least 3–5 min.

Alternative to 7.1: With TIVA, but without TCI, without nitrous oxide

This alternative is similar to recipe 7.1 with the exception of the following paragraphs:

Induction

a. Use one iv line (dorsum of hand or crook of elbow), run in Ringer's solution for induction, one-way valves, and three-way couplings (see Figure 7.1). Start with propofol 20 mg bolus and 2 mg/kg per hour for sedation as soon as is feasible. Put on ECG, BP cuff, pulse oximeter, and note baseline values.

b. **Induction**: propofol bolus 1.5 mg/kg, then infusion at 10 mg/kg per hour, then immediately start remifentanil infusion 0.6 µg/kg per minute if LMA is planned, or 0.8 µg/kg per minute if endotracheal tube is planned. (If the patient is > 60 years I reduce the remifentanil dose by 10–50%.) Ask the patient to breathe oxygen deeply by mask; assist as needed.
   After 2–3 min the patient's jaw feels relaxed and the LMA or endotracheal tube may be inserted.

c. Insert the LMA or endotracheal tube.

d. Turn propofol down to 8 mg/kg per hour 10 min after the start; then turn it down to 6 mg/kg per hour 20 min after the start. Turn remifentanil down to 0.2 µg/kg per minute while waiting for surgery to start and then up to 0.4–0.6 µg/kg per hour 1 min before surgery starts, depending upon the anticipated strength of surgical stimulation.

Maintenance

a. Keep propofol at 6 mg/kg per hour as a baseline drug for sleep. Adjust between 4 and 8 mg/kg per hour according to the case. Do not let it fall below 4 mg/kg per hour, otherwise sudden emergence may occur. Occasionally increase it to 8 mg/kg per minute (perhaps with a 0.5 mg/kg bolus first) if the patient opens their eyes or moves despite a low BP, low heart rate, and adequate remifentanil level. Try to adjust the propofol level down to 4–5 mg/kg per hour during the last 10 min.

b. Remifentanil should be adjusted freely according to the patient's sensitivity and strength of surgical stimulation; anything from 0.2 to 0.8 (or even 1.0) µg/kg per minute as needed.

Alternative to 7.3: With TIVA, without TCI, supplemented with nitrous oxide

This alternative is similar to recipe 7.3 with the exception of the following paragraphs:

Induction

d. Start nitrous oxide; 4 l/min in 2 l/min oxygen; after 10 min turn down nitrous oxide to 2 l/min and oxygen to 1 l/min if you have a circulating ventilator system with a scavenger. Otherwise, maintain levels at 4+2 l/min.

e. Turn propofol down to 6 mg/kg per hour once nitrous oxide is started and then down to 4 mg/kg per hour 5 min later. Turn remifentanil down to 0.2 μg/kg per minute while waiting for surgery to start, and then up to 0.4–0.6 μg/kg per hour 1 min before the start of surgery.

   If the patient did not receive paracetamol or NSAID/COX-II inhibitor tablets for premedication, then give paracetamol 1 g as an iv infusion. If there is no risk of bleeding, give ketorolac 30 mg as the NSAID; if there is a risk of bleeding (or conventional NSAID is inferior in other aspects) I give either parecoxib 40 mg or I wait until hemostasis is ensured before giving ketorolac.

Maintenance

b. Keep propofol in the 3–4 mg/kg per hour range as a baseline drug for sleep together with nitrous oxide. Do not let it fall below 3 mg/kg per hour, otherwise sudden emergence may occur. Raise the propofol to 6 mg/kg at the start if the patient opens their eyes or moves despite a low BP, low heart rate, and adequate remifentanil level.

End of case

d. Turn the TCI of propofol and remifentanil to zero.
   Turn nitrous oxide to zero, and the oxygen rate to 6 l/min.

Mixed iv anesthesia with inhalational anesthesia maintenance

Indicated when propofol or remifentanil infusion for maintenance is not used.

   The sequence is the same as for *propofol and remifentanil* as in recipe 7.1 until the LMA or endotracheal tube is in place. Then start with either sevoflurane 2–8% (1–2 MAC) or desflurane 4–6% (0.5–1 MAC). Desflurane should be introduced slowly, as a sudden start with more than 1–2 MAC may induce sympathetic stimulation. Then adjust the vaporizer settings according to end-tidal measurements, to the fresh gas flow, and to the level of surgical stress and opioid. Turn the propofol off. If there is an option to use remifentanil throughout the case, I opt for a baseline sleeping dose of inhalational agent at about 0.5–1.0 MAC (adjust for age) and then use remifentanil as the analgesic component as needed. If the case is longer than 1–2 h, if the patient is obese, or if the patient is a child, I prefer to use desflurane if there is a choice; otherwise, sevoflurane does very well.

Propofol and fentanyl opioid bolus start and supplements

Premedication and use of NSAID/COX-II inhibitor are as in recipe 7.1.

Induction

a. Use one iv line (dorsum of hand or crook of elbow), run Ringer's solution for induction, hub or three-way valve for syringe injections. Start with propofol 20 mg bolus and perhaps 10 mg as needed if the patient is very anxious when arriving in theater (otherwise skip this).

    Put on ECG, BP cuff, and pulse oximeter, and note baseline values.

b. **Induction**: propofol bolus 2 mg/kg, then the opioid, e.g., fentanyl right away, 100–200 μg. After 2–3 min this will usually do for LMA insertion.

c. Put in the LMA. If the patient needs intubating then a neuromuscular blocking agent should preferably be used, otherwise the extra dose of opioid has to be quite high – alfentanil 2–3 mg or fentanyl 200–300 μg timed appropriately before intubation.

Maintenance

Give fentanyl again, 100–200 μg, when surgery starts and then 100 μg every 30–60 min as needed. Without propofol infusion the patient will need inhalational maintenance to keep them asleep – either a potent agent in combination with nitrous oxide or a potent agent alone. The total MAC should be in the range 0.5–1.0 to ensure the patient stays asleep. The fentanyl schedule above may result in prolonged emergence, thus it may be helpful to reduce the need for fentanyl once the LMA is in place by using nitrous oxide, sevoflurane, or desflurane at an end-tidal MAC value of 1–2 to provide additional antinociceptive effect from the gas. Alternatively one may do without further fentanyl, in which case one must be prepared to use inhalational agents in the 1.5–3.0 MAC range.

Propofol and alfentanil opioid bolus start and supplements

Premedication and use of NSAID/COX-II inhibitor as in recipe 7.1.

Induction

a. Use one iv line (dorsum of hand or crook of elbow), run Ringer's solution for induction, hub or three-way valve for syringe injections. Start with propofol 20 mg bolus and perhaps 10 mg as needed if the patient is very anxious when arriving in theater (otherwise skip).

    Put on ECG, BP cuff, and pulse oximeter, and note baseline values.

b. **Induction**: propofol bolus 2 mg/kg, then wait 1 min and give alfentanil, 1.0–2.0 mg.

    Waiting 1–2 min usually suffices for LMA insertion.

c. Put in the LMA (or intubate, see above).

Maintenance

Give alfentanil again, 0.5–1.5 mg, when surgery starts, and then 0.5 mg every 15–30 min as needed. Without propofol infusion the patient will need inhalational maintenance to be kept asleep: either a potent agent in combination with nitrous oxide or a potent agent alone. The total MAC should be in the 0.5–1.0 range to keep the patient asleep. The alfentanil schedule above is not liable to prolong emergence, nevertheless it may be helpful to reduce the need for alfentanil once the LMA is in place by using nitrous oxide, sevoflurane, or desflurane at an end-tidal MAC value of 1–2 to provide additional antinociceptive effect from the gas. Alternatively, one may do without further alfentanil, in which case one must be prepared to use inhalational agents in the 1.5–3.0 MAC range.

Propofol and fentanyl + alfentanil opioid technique

As fentanyl is a slow drug with prolonged elimination compared with alfentanil, it may be wise to combine these opioids in order to ensure a stable baseline and appropriate post-operative analgesia (fentanyl) with the benefit of the strong and short-lasting adjunct from alfentanil.

Induction

a. Use one iv line (dorsum of hand or crook of the elbow), run Ringer's solution for induction, hub or three-way valve for syringe injections. Start with propofol 20 mg bolus and perhaps 10 mg as needed if the patient is very anxious when arriving in theater (otherwise skip).

    Put on ECG, BP cuff, and pulse oximeter, and note baseline values.

b. **Induction**: propofol bolus 2 mg/kg and fentanyl 100 μg; then wait 1 min and give alfentanil, 1.0 mg. (If intubating without curare, alfentanil 2.0–3.0 mg.)

    Waiting 1–2 min usually suffices for LMA insertion.

c. Put in the LMA (or intubate, see above).

Maintenance

Give alfentanil again, 0.5–1.5 mg, when surgery starts, and then 0.5 mg every 15–30 min as needed. Without propofol infusion the patient will need inhalational maintenance to be kept asleep; either a potent agent in combination with nitrous oxide or a potent agent alone. The total MAC should be in the 0.5–1.0 range to keep the patient asleep. The fentanyl + alfentanil schedule above is not liable to prolong emergence, nevertheless it may be helpful to reduce the need for alfentanil once the LMA is in place by using nitrous oxide, or sevoflurane, or desflurane at an end-tidal MAC value of 1–2 to provide additional antinociceptive effect from the gas. Alternatively, one may do without further alfentanil, in which case one must be prepared to use inhalational agents in the 1.5–3.0 MAC range.

5–10 min before the end of the procedure: fentanyl 100 μg.

Inhalational induction, adults

In some adults it may be better to do a mask induction; for instance, if the patient is hard or impossible to communicate with (psychiatric condition, dementia, brain damage) and strongly resists any attempt at venous stasis or needle insertion. There are also patients who are otherwise competent but have a strong needle phobia. If these patients cannot be convinced about the benefits of EMLA® cream and painless cannulation, they should be offered the choice of induction by mask using sevoflurane.

My technique is simply to have the patient breathing 100% oxygen by mask for 10–15 s, and then turn on 8% sevoflurane and maintain this until they are asleep, maybe with gentle bag and mask assistance. As they fall asleep some patients may become a little agitated or hyperventilate (and often have diverging eyes) before their facial muscles relax and their

Table 7.1. Neuromuscular blocking agents

Drug	Dose (mg/kg)	Onset[a](s)	Duration[b] (min)	Supplement (% of)	Elimination	Indication
Suxamethonium	1	55	10		Plasma cholinesterase	RSI
Rocuronium	0.6	75	30	20–30	Liver	RSI Elective surgery
Vecuronium	0.1	120	30	20–30	Liver, kidney	Elective surgery (RSI)
Cisatracurium	0.15	180	50	20–30	Liver + spontaneous degradation	Elective surgery Organ failure
Mivacurium	0.2	180[c]	15	50 (5–10 µg/kg per minute)	Plasma cholinesterase	Short procedures

RSI, Rapid-sequence induction.
[a] Monitoring of effect in m. adductor pollicis.
[b] Duration: Time from injection to new dose needed, i.e., TOF: 2–4 twitches.
[c] Intubation after 120 s.

breathing becomes even and shallow. At this point an iv cannula should be inserted, and I then continue with one of the intravenous techniques described above. The only difference is that I halve the initial propofol bolus, but target everything else the same.

Adding neuromuscular blocking agent (NMBA)

See 4.2.5 Neuromuscular blockers and reversal agents for details of indication and drugs.

The dosing in Table 7.1 is for achieving a 90–100% block, which may be needed for some types of microsurgery where the patient should remain 100% immobile, e.g., some types of eye surgery, middle ear surgery, plastic surgery, or microsurgery.

In these cases, the train-of-four (TOF) twitches should be kept at 0–1 at all times.

For most other elective indications of NMBA the starting dose may be set at about 50% of the values in Table 7.1, with a TOF of 2–3 twitches. Under these circumstances good relaxation is achieved but the patient is still able to move if they experience discomfort (awareness protection) and the neuromuscular block can be easily reversed at the end of surgery.

Special procedures and/or patients
Children

My usual choice is to skip anxiolytic premedication. If the child is very anxious or stressed, midazolam (0.25–0.5 mg/kg) may be given orally 45–60 min beforehand. If the child is willing to take tablets 1–2 h before surgery, I give analgesic prophylaxis: paracetamol 25–40 mg/kg and diclofenac 1–1.5 mg/kg. EMLA® pads should be applied to the dorsum of both hands at least 45–60 min before induction is due to start. Most parents are able to apply the pads before leaving home if they are sent proper instructions. Extra taping or wearing gloves are some tricks that can be used to keep the pads on an active child.

The induction should be carried out with minimal "fuss"; for example, allow the child to keep their normal indoor clothes on, and sit them on their parent's knee. Have the induction drugs ready, and insert a 0.8 mm venous cannula and immediately connect it to Ringer's acetate solution (500 ml bag, as a 1000 ml bag is risky if everything runs in quickly). Use a pulse oximeter as the only monitoring; no preoxygenation.

Induction is with propofol 4–5 mg/kg (max. 150 mg) and alfentanil 25 µg/kg (the propofol is pretreated by adding 1 mg/ml lidocaine). When the child falls asleep, immediately position them on the table and start mask ventilation with 100% oxygen. At this point the parents should leave the room. ECG and blood-pressure cuff are put on (may be skipped in very short cases of 5–10 min) and the child is given dexamethasone 0.2–0.5 mg/kg (usual standard dose is 4 mg). If they have not received paracetamol beforehand, they will be given 50 mg/kg (40–60 mg range) rectally and perhaps diclofenac 2 mg/kg via the same route. As COX inhibitors are not yet approved for children, this is not an option; thus if there are potential problems of bleeding or hemostasis, NSAIDs should not be given until after the operation.

The routine with children is then to insert the LMA, or with a short procedure just do mask ventilation.

This induction will usually do for 5–10 min of maintenance; after that supplements of propofol 0.5 mg/kg and alfentanil 10 mg/kg may be given every 5 min (or every 10 min with use of nitrous oxide). The surgeon should be encouraged to use local anesthesia infiltration. With procedures in the genital and perineal areas or for inguinal hernia, a caudal block may be very effective for postoperative pain control.

If postoperative pain is expected to be strong, fentanyl 0.5 µg/kg may be given at the end of the procedure.

With procedures lasting longer than 15–20 min it is more practical to continue with either propofol + remifentanil infusions or with inhalational anesthesia.

Propofol + remifentanil infusion – TCI or infusion

With remifentanil the same dosing and strategies can be used as in adults, maybe with slightly higher target values (+10–20%).

With propofol a child TCI algorithm should be used, either the Paedfusor® or the Kataria® model, which both integrate a higher initial volume of distribution (V1) and clearance in children. With these models the targets should be about 10–20% higher than for adults; if manual dosing is selected then the bolus should be about 50–100% higher than for adults per kilogram (i.e., 3–5 mg/kg) and maintenance about 25–50% higher.

Inhalational maintenance

With inhalational maintenance the same MAC values as for adults may be used, but the dosing of MAC should be age-adjusted. The additive effect of 67% nitrous oxide in children is 0.3–0.4 MAC and not 0.5 MAC as in adults.

It is wise to use local anesthesia generously as with TIVA techniques and if emergence pain is expected, supplement with fentanyl 0.5 µg/kg at the end of surgery.

The ENT child

Myringotomy

For these patients I use propofol + alfentanil induction (see above) and maintain assisted face mask ventilation. If a top-up is needed, I give more alfentanil or use a 1MAC dose of sevoflurane.

Adenoidectomy and tonsillectomy

I prefer to intubate these patients with the regime below as it avoids delays and problems with airway control. For the adenoids I use an uncuffed tube, whereas for tonsillectomies I like to have the option of protecting the airway from blood by having a cuffed tube. The idea is not to fill the cuff, but just have it there as an option in the rare case of a significant bleed.

Many units use the LMA for these cases if the surgeon is experienced.

After induction (alfentanil + propofol) I spray the trachea and vocal cords with lidocaine 40 mg/ml, 0.1 ml/kg and then ventilate with oxygen by mask for 1 min and intubate.

The surgeon should be urged to infiltrate the tonsil beds with local anesthesia for better postoperative analgesia.

After emergence there should be a low threshold for giving fentanyl 0.5 µg/kg iv for pain.

Ketamine sedation in children

For procedures with no or limited surgical stimulation (X-ray, diagnostic procedures), a simplified sedation regime of ketamine + midazolam works very well with a spontaneously breathing child with an unassisted free airway and stable hemodynamics.

The baseline medication is midazolam 0.1 mg/kg iv, and then ketamine 1 mg/kg iv. No further midazolam is given, but ketamine is given as required in 1 mg/kg supplements, usually every 10–30 min depending upon stimulation.

Monitor with pulse oximetry and give extra oxygen (mask or nasal catheter) if needed (if saturation falls below 92%).

Laparoscopy

Due to routine use of a gastric tube, oral preoperative pain medication is skipped. My preference is to use TIVA with propofol + remifentanil for these patients, and usually no neuromuscular blocking agent (except in very obese patients or when the surgeon requests it) and an LMA with a gastric tube in place (e.g., ProSeal™).

As the pressure in the abdomen is liable to change abruptly, volume-controlled ventilator mode is optimal as in pressure-control mode an increase in abdominal pressure may lead to hypoventilation that is overlooked. Also, PEEP (4 cmH$_2$O, or 6 cmH$_2$O in the obese) is useful in order to minimize microatelectasis in the lung bases.

With laparoscopy an optimal nonopioid and anti-emetic regimen is very important and my routine is as follows:

- **Analgesia (present at emergence):**
  - bupivacaine/ropivacaine wound infiltration
  - paracetamol 1.0 g iv
  - ketorolac (NSAID) 20–30 mg iv (or parecoxib, see NSAID)
  - dexamethasone 8 mg iv
  - fentanyl 1–2 µg/kg at the end of surgery
- **Anti-emesis:**
  - droperidol 1.25 mg iv
  - (dexamethasone, also given for pain)
  - ondansetron 4 mg iv
  - propofol anesthesia + remifentanil anesthesia, no nitrous oxide, low opioid hangover

Dental surgery

Dental surgery will most often be done under local anesthesia, perhaps with mild general sedation from benzodiazepines administered by the dentist or dental surgeon. However, some patients have "dentophobia" and need either professional sedation (see Chapter 5) or general anesthesia for the procedure.

Propofol-induced sleep is a very good basis for dental anesthesia, but also low-dose (0.5–0.75 MAC) desflurane inhalation may be excellent in very prolonged cases where a rapid and clearheaded recovery is important. The base hypnotic agent should be supplemented with generous and adequate local anesthesia administered by the dentist or dental surgeon. Extra opioid is still required, during the injection of local anesthesia, at painful parts of surgery and due to irritation from the laryngeal mask or the stronger irritation of an endotracheal tube. Particularly painful moments may be treated with injection of 0.5 mg alfentanil as needed (or remifentanil 0.5–1.0 µg/kg), whereas a more continuous need for basic opioid effect may be achieved with remifentanil infusion (0.1–0.3 µg/kg per minute or target 2.5–7.5 ng/ml) or small doses of fentanyl 0.5–1.0 µg/kg every 30–60 min.

An important issue to clarify is whether the dental surgeon can work with an LMA or whether intubation is needed. An endotracheal tube is less bulky than an LMA, does not become dislodged, and will protect the airway better against micro-aspiration, especially if the cuff is sealed and a cotton dressing swab is placed in the pharynx together with a suction device. A nasotracheal tube provides the best working conditions for the surgeon, but always carries a small risk of nasal bleeding and an even smaller risk of sinusitis. It is definitely worth while spending the extra money on a soft-walled tube, and also to use a topical vasoconstrictor and a gel lubricant in the nostril before insertion. However, for many procedures surgeons will be able to work with an oral tube in place. This may be sited in one corner of the mouth at the start and then moved to the other corner during the procedure to allow the surgeon access to all areas.

Eye surgery

Eye surgery can mostly be done under local anesthesia or an eye block, but children and some adults require general anesthesia. For many procedures an LMA technique is acceptable, but should be weighed against the difficulties in each case of getting access to the airways in case of dislodgement.

Some eye surgeons will routinely ask for 100% muscle relaxation; this can be queried for many types of eye surgery as the surgeon usually sees (and communicates!) small, innocent papillary or eye muscle reactions that occur before there is any danger of gross movements.

Orthopedic surgery

Orthopedic procedures causing trauma to bones and tissue structures are usually accompanied by substantial pain afterwards and for this reason loco-regional techniques should be given serious consideration, perhaps supplemented with propofol sedation or propofol + remifentanil anesthesia and LMA. For minor traumatic procedures, such as diagnostic arthroscopies, a general anesthetic technique may save time and be easily adjusted with local anesthesia if the procedure becomes more extensive.

Obese patients (see also The obese patient)

These patients should have standard monitoring with ECG, noninvasive blood pressure measurement, pulse oximetry, nerve stimulation test of neuromuscular block (i.e., TOF guard®), end-tidal CO_2 measurement, and anesthetic gas analysis. An arterial line for invasive blood pressure measurement is only inserted if specifically indicated, e.g., patients with known cardiovascular problems.

It may be useful to monitor the depth of anesthesia in these patients, but this may be skipped during inhalational-based anesthesia if end-tidal MAC values are above 1 MAC all the time.

Our recipe for obese patients undergoing laparoscopy is as follows:

- When preoxygenation is fulfilled, anesthesia is induced with propofol and remifentanil plasma target controlled infusions (TCI) with targets of 6 µg/ml and 8 ng/ml, respectively. Both infusions are based on corrected ideal weight (height in centimeters minus 100, plus 20% of the difference between the real weight and ideal weight).

- Then, vecuronium 0.08 mg/kg corrected ideal weight is given.

- Tracheal intubation is performed with the patient in the semi-sitting position with their neck flexed on the trunk and the head extended on the neck ("sniffing the morning air" position). A standard laryngoscope with a short handle and an endotracheal tube with a stylet are used.

- After the tracheal tube is secured, the propofol infusion is stopped and inhalation of desflurane at 3–6% (i.e., 0.5–1 MAC) is started. Inspiratory oxygen is reduced to 40% and PEEP to 5 cmH$_2$O.

- A gastric tube is inserted and the gastric content (if any) is aspirated.

- Anesthesia is continued throughout the operation with remifentanil and desflurane. The doses are adjusted according to clinical observation, arterial blood pressure, and bispectral index (BIS). Typically, remifentanil TCI is adjusted within a wide range to keep systolic blood pressure within acceptable limits (i.e., 85–120 mmHg) and desflurane is adjusted to keep the BIS within the range of 45–55.

- Droperidol 1.25 mg, ondansetron 4 mg, and dexamethasone 8 mg are given as routine iv anti-emetic prophylaxis.

- Parecoxib 40 mg, paracetamol 1 g iv, and bupivacaine 5 mg/ml around the incisions, in a total volume of 30–40 ml, are given to prevent postoperative pain. Furthermore, fentanyl 100 µg is given before the end of surgery.

- Desflurane and remifentanil are stopped upon removal of the laparoscope at the end of surgery, and a small dose of propofol (30–50 mg total) is then given. The neuromuscular block is reversed with neostigmine 2.5 mg and glycopyrrolate 1 mg and the patients are ventilated with 100% oxygen. The patients are extubated on the table when they are emerging, breathing, and showing the first signs of irritation from the tracheal tube. Then patients move themselves, with some assistance, into the bed.

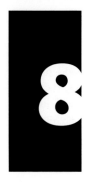

8 Some controversies in ambulatory anesthesia

Total intravenous anesthesia or inhalational anesthesia for ambulatory care?

The clinical issues to focus on when choosing an anesthetic technique are: rapid induction, smooth maintenance, rapid emergence, and adequate pain control, so that after the procedure the patients are fully awake and not suffering side-effects such as nausea, vomiting, and shivering.

When general anesthesia is provided with intravenous agents alone, this is called total intravenous anesthesia (TIVA, see also Chapter 4, Pharmacology). The characteristics of TIVA compared with alternative techniques (i.e., loco-regional anesthesia, inhalational anesthesia) concern not only the concept per se but also the characteristics of the drugs used.

The TIVA concept is simple. An intravenous line is the only prerequisite, and everything needed for general anesthesia is supplied through this line, obviating the need for sophisticated gas delivery systems and scavenger equipment. The alternatives of regional blocks or neuraxial blocks take more time to establish. There is no risk of block failure or problems caused by the unpredictable duration of residual paralysis.

The TIVA drugs are generally less toxic than inhalational agents, have less risk of causing malignant hyperthermia, and do not pollute the environmental air or atmosphere. TIVA usually necessitates component therapy, with different drugs dedicated to achieving different effects; typically one drug for the hypnotic effect (propofol, ketamine, methohexital, midazolam), and another for analgesia and antinociception (remifentanil, other opioids, ketamine).

TIVA versus nitrous oxide supplementation

In most reviews nitrous oxide is associated with an increased risk of postoperative nausea and vomiting (PONV) [1]. This was recently confirmed in a large study of more than 2000 inpatients by Leslie et al. [2]. However, in a study of ambulatory orthopedic patients, Mathews et al. found no significant side-effects of nitrous oxide when compared with remifentanil as an adjunct to general anesthesia. The time to emergence was also similar in the two groups [3]. Nitrous oxide is associated with rapid emergence and has a minor influence on respiratory function, and may be used as an adjunct to reduce the dose of propofol needed. In a study of oocyte retrieval, Handa-Tsutsui and Kodaka found a 20% reduction in dose of propofol needed when nitrous oxide was used, without any obvious clinical benefits or drawbacks [4].

TIVA versus inhalational anesthesia

Inhalational anesthesia usually implies inhalational maintenance, with or without opioid supplementation, after an intravenous induction. In a study of septorhinoplasty Gokce et al. [5] did not find any significant differences between desflurane + remifentanil maintenance versus propofol + remifentanil. In a more detailed study of microsurgical vertebral disk resection, Gozdemir et al. found shorter emergence and less nausea, but more shivering and postoperative pain in the propofol + remifentanil group, when compared with the desflurane + nitrous oxide group [6]. Increased incidence of postoperative shivering was also found after remifentanil + propofol in Röhm et al.'s comparison with desflurane + fentanyl [7]. Moore et al. confirmed the well-known benefit of reduced PONV after TIVA with propofol in mixed-case day surgery [8]. Similarly, reduced PONV was found by Hong et al. after breast biopsy with propofol + remifentanil anesthesia [9]. However, their result may be biased by the use of a longer-acting opioid, fentanyl, in the control group. Inhalational induction with sevoflurane + nitrous oxide was slower, but smoother (i.e., less bradycardia and apnea) and associated with slower emergence and less postoperative pain compared to the TIVA technique in this study [9]. In a large study of 1158 adults in ambulatory mixed surgery, Moore et al. compared different methods of sevoflurane with/without nitrous oxide induction and/ or maintenance versus propofol TIVA [8]. They found more injection pain and hiccups with propofol and more breath-holding and recalled discomfort with sevoflurane induction. Sevoflurane was associated with more PONV, but the major outcome results, such as time to discharge and unplanned hospital admissions, were similar in both groups [8].

The problem of coughing during emergence and extubation was addressed specifically in a study of lumbar disk surgery by Hohlrieder et al. [10]. They found significantly less coughing when propofol + remifentanil was compared with sevoflurane + nitrous oxide + fentanyl. Aspects of early and late PONV were addressed by White et al. in a study of day-case gynecologic surgery [11]. They report similar predischarge PONV incidence when dolasetron was added to sevoflurane maintenance and compared with propofol + remifentanil. However, as discussed by the authors, the dolasetron effect is prolonged compared with propofol, explaining why the dolasetron + sevoflurane patients had less PONV after discharge [11].

Gastric emptying may also have an impact on PONV incidence. This was investigated by Walldén et al. in a study of ambulatory laparoscopic cholecystectomies [12]. They found a generally delayed and variable gastric emptying rate in their patients, but no difference between the propofol + remifentanil group and the sevoflurane group [12].

As inhalational agents may be used in low-flow re-breathing systems, they may be more cost-effective than propofol. This was demonstrated in a study of sevoflurane + sufentanil versus propofol + sufentanil for laparoscopic cholecystectomy [13].

There have been some reports on sevoflurane-induced convulsions [14] and potentially negative effects in brain trauma patients [15], but these concerns do not seem to be very relevant to ambulatory procedures. Similarly, the benefits of preconditioning and protection against cardiac ischemia with inhalational agents have not yet been demonstrated to be of clinical importance in ambulatory surgery, and may be disputed even for major surgery [16]. More clinically important are the reports of emergence agitation in children, which are more frequent after sevoflurane anesthesia than propofol [17].

Drugs and adjuncts in TIVA

In many places the combination of propofol and remifentanil is synonymous with TIVA. Both drugs are supplied as a continuous infusion. Propofol may be titrated against an EEG-based hypnotic monitor (e.g., BIS or other) or kept at a fairly constant level for assuring sleep, whereas the remifentanil delivery may be adjusted more frequently and vigorously according to surgical stimulation and nociceptive input.

Methohexital is a cheaper alternative to propofol, and was recently compared with propofol or midazolam for oral and maxillofacial surgery [18]. The methohexital patients had more adverse events, especially nausea. Propofol was better in this respect, also when compared to midazolam.

As pump technology is expensive, there may still be an option for ketamine as a single all-purpose drug in settings of limited resources [19]. Ketamine is traditionally associated with slower emergence and some incidence of unpleasant hallucinations even when given in moderate doses for sedation [20]. However, Friedberg et al. have repeatedly reported a high success rate for ketamine sedation during plastic surgery under local anesthesia. Propofol with increasing supplement of ketamine for light or profound sedation during spontaneous ventilation gave no hallucinations and virtually no PONV [21,22]. Recent publications in the ambulatory setting partly support this conclusion [23,24]. However, Aouad et al. reported more agitation [25], Goel et al. reported delayed recovery [26], and a review from Slavik and Zed concluded that there are no specific benefits with this technique [27]. Interest has also been shown in low-dose ketamine infusion for the reduction of postoperative pain and hyperalgesia [28]. However, the clinical relevance of this, if any, needs to be further tested in ambulatory anesthesia.

The use of neuromuscular blocking agents (NMBA) seems to be declining in ambulatory care, also when endotracheal intubation is used. Gravningsbråten et al. [29] did not use NMBAs for ENT surgery and Paek et al. [30] did without them for intubation in laparoscopic surgery without any problems. However, intubation without muscle relaxants requires a high dose of opioid to be successful. Thus some cases of severe hypotension may be seen, especially in old, fragile patients. Injury of the vocal cords has been described after intubation without NMBA, but clinical studies have not been able to show fewer symptoms of airway trauma with curare than without [31,32].

A beta-blocker is an adjunct that is strongly recommended for surgery in patients with coronary disease, although its perioperative benefits in beta-blocker-naive patients are disputed and controversial [33]. Beta-blockers will stabilize the hemodynamics during surgery [34], but may also have other interesting effects in ambulatory surgery. In a study of cholecystectomies, Collard et al. used esmolol infusion instead of opioids, i.e., remifentanil or fentanyl, during laparoscopic surgery [35]. The results are remarkable, as the beneficial effects of beta-blocker were evident throughout early recovery: less nausea, less pain, and more rapid discharge [35].

Development of TIVA

The future of TIVA may change, as a result of both upcoming new drugs and more sophisticated delivery and monitoring equipment.

In most countries, target control systems for TIVA have been launched. Initially, only the Diprifusor® with the Marsh pharmacokinetic model for plasma propofol was available. Now, open target control infusion (TCI) systems are available from many manufacturers, and there is a choice of different dosing models for propofol, remifentanil, and other opioids. The idea of TCI is to deliver drug intravenously to maintain a precise drug level, either in the plasma (plasma TCI) or at the brain effect site (effect-site TCI). The drug is infused automatically from a pump programmed with the patient's data (e.g., weight, height, age). The anesthesiologist may adjust target levels according to variable clinical need during the procedure [36]. Also, new monitoring devices are being introduced, in which the combined anesthetic effect of different TIVA drugs is simulated, added, and displayed on the monitor [37]. A further development of TCI is the automatic, closed-loop system that incorporates the information provided by EEG or auditory evoked potential (AEP) and hemodynamics monitoring to adjust the TCI pumps automatically. Successful reports of such systems are emerging [38–40]. Such systems may simplify dosing further, but they all involve a delay from clinical response to dose adjustment, and will certainly never be able to predict increased dose need in anticipation of especially painful parts of surgery.

Dexmedetomidine has already been launched in many countries as a promising analgesic and anxiolytic drug for sedation, for minor procedures in children, and intensive care settings [41]. The potential of dexmedetomidine in ambulatory general anesthesia is also being explored, but so far the prolonged recovery after the high doses needed for anesthesia compared with propofol appear to be a clinical limitation [42,43]. However, as the need for opioid may be reduced or even eliminated with dexmedetomidine the incidence of PONV is also reduced. This point was shown in a study of laparoscopy with dexmedetomidine + desflurane by Salman et al. [43].

Propofol 5 mg/ml has recently been introduced and found to cause less aching during induction in children compared with the present dose of 10 mg/ml, both dissolved in mixed long- and medium-chain triglyceride (solution) [44]. A prodrug of propofol, fospropofol, has been launched as a water-soluble alternative for sedation, but the prolonged induction time and increased amount of vein pain during induction may limit its potential to replace propofol [45]. The ongoing attempts to make an esterase-degraded, ultra-short-acting propofol analog may be more interesting, but so far the trials for this drug (THRX-918661) have not been published. Results from animal studies of the new, short-acting, esterase-degraded benzodiazepine (CNS-7056) seem very promising [46]. The first human clinical study is in progress and seems to confirm an ultra-short duration combined with otherwise traditional benzodiazepine characteristics (G. Kilpatrick, personal communication).

Benefits of inhalational anesthesia

The inhalational agents are amnesic and hypnotic agents used in low doses (at MAC levels 0.5–1.0) with increasing antinociceptive, analgesic effect as the dosing is increased. As they are exhaled at the end of anesthesia, they have organ-independent elimination. They are very safe in the multi-allergic patients, and drug waste at the end of a case is minimal, as surplus drug in the vaporizer is used for the next case. Drug economy may be very good if a low-flow system of fresh gas is used, but expensive if a high-flow system with any of the newer agents is used.

Although some pulmonary shunting disturbs the equilibration between alveoli and mixed arterial blood, the option of using end-tidal measurements to provide an online indication of anesthetic drug level in the individual patient is not yet available for intravenous drugs. Clinically, the inhalational agents are not as strongly respiratory depressant as a combined opioid + propofol technique, and for that reason they are more successful if spontaneous ventilation is required.

Inhalational induction in ambulatory care

This remains the preferred method of many anesthesiologists for children, as no establishment of an iv line is needed first. The child may sit on their parent's knee and spontaneously breathe sevoflurane 8% in oxygen or oxygen/air. Some prefer to start with nitrous oxide, while others like to introduce the nitrous oxide after a few breaths of sevoflurane in order to have a secondary gas effect from the increasing concentration of sevoflurane in the alveoli as the nitrous oxide is absorbed extensively into the blood. Even without nitrous oxide the induction is usually smooth, occurring within 1–2 min, and the child may be managed further with an iv line, iv drugs, or by continuing with the inhalational technique alone. Halothane may be an alternative for smooth induction, although the emergence may be delayed. Desflurane and isoflurane are generally considered unsuitable for inhalational induction as they are very irritant and dosing must be increased slowly in order to avoid coughing, hiccups, and even laryngospasm.

Inhalational induction may also be an option in adults, if there is a special request or if the patient has a needle phobia. Sometimes for psychiatric patients or patients with impaired cognitive function, it may be preferable to avoid needles.

One problem with inhalational induction is the absence of an iv line, which is required if the patient suddenly becomes hypotensive, bradycardic, or has a bronchial spasm during induction. The anesthesiologist should prepare for such potential problems by having suxamethonium ready for intramuscular (tongue is best!) injection as well as some vasopressor to hand.

Inhalational maintenance and ending of the case

As quite high concentrations may be needed in order to blunt strong surgical stimulation when given alone, inhalational agents may be combined with opioid analgesics in order to keep the dose at a level that ensures sleep alone. Both enflurane and desflurane are associated with a slightly more rapid emergence than propofol, and may be easier to dose, especially in the elderly, the obese, patients with drug abuse problems, or those with abnormal iv drug degradation.

For prolonged procedures (i.e., more than 2–3 h) the emergence after desflurane will be slightly faster because it is less soluble in tissue compared with sevoflurane. This difference is more pronounced in the obese, where a more rapid desflurane recovery may be seen also after procedures lasting 1–2 h. Another problem with sevoflurane is the high incidence of emergence agitation seen in children. As this incidence is lower with desflurane, some authors recommend switching to desflurane after a sevoflurane induction. Also, Einarsson et al. have demonstrated that desflurane is less of a respiratory depressant at equipotent concentrations [47]. While most studies show that inhalational agents result in more PONV than propofol-based techniques, the issue of shivering is more controversial. It seems that isoflurane is worse than other agents in terms of normothermic shivering [48], but studies with the new inhalational agents suggest otherwise, i.e., that sevoflurane and desflurane may result in less shivering than propofol [6,7].

Do we need "depth of anesthesia" monitoring in ambulatory anesthesia?

The idea of "depth-of-anesthesia-monitoring" (DAM) is to provide an evaluation of the pharmacologic effect of anesthetic drugs that is more accurate and precise than end-tidal monitoring of gases or simulation of iv plasma levels. DAM should also be more sensitive and specific than the clinical monitoring of effects, such as sympathomimetic output, hemodynamics, and movements. As it is potentially harmful to have a level of anesthesia that is either too light or too deep, it is a good idea to provide some "warning" of clinical changes in either direction. The two indications for DAM are prevention of awareness (i.e., underdosing) and more precise titration of the correct drug dose (i.e., over- or underdosing).

There are numerous commercial methods and devices for DAM [49]. Many use the recorded EEG, whereas others use the EEG response to a stimulus. These methods are depth-of-sleep monitors, but there are other devices that attempt to measure the nociception-induced stress level, by using the R-R interval in ECG, muscle tension, pulse amplitude, or sweating [50]. The most-used and best-documented device is the BIS monitor, which transforms a passive, sampled frontal EEG and compares it using an algorithm with a "data bank" of empirical EEG patterns [51]. The BIS is calibrated to give a signal of 0–100, where values below 60 indicate unconsciousness or sleep in most patients. Keeping the BIS value in the 40–60 range (or even better 50–60 range) during general anesthesia ensures rapid emergence and less risk of overdosing in individual patients. Shortcomings with BIS include the inability to account for the influence of opioid or nitrous oxide supplements, and a paradoxical increase in the BIS value when ketamine is given to a sleeping patient.

Awareness is quite rare, about 1 per 500 in newer studies without DAM [52]. Unpleasant awareness only occurs in fully curarized patients, because noncurarized patients will move if they are uncomfortable and are becoming aware. In order to be aware it seems that a period of at least 4 min of BIS above 60 is needed [52]. It has been shown in two studies, one in high-risk procedures (mostly emergency) [53] and the other in inhalational-based inpatient anesthesia [52], that awareness is significantly reduced by 80% if BIS monitoring is used. The cost-benefit relevance of these studies for ambulatory cases is disputed, as deep curarization is infrequent and the costs of BIS electrodes range from 10–15 euro per case. It has also been claimed that, with inhalational anesthesia, keeping the end-tidal gas level at appropriate values (1 MAC or more) may be as sensitive and as specific as BIS monitoring for avoiding reaction and awareness [54]. BIS values above 60 for more than 4 min happens in about 20% of cases, and only 1 out of 500 of these will be aware [52]. Where the BIS is observed to be above 60 drugs may be dosed more generously; therefore, overall the costs of implementing procedures to avoid just one case of awareness are quite high. Nevertheless, if economy permits, it may be a good choice in terms of the patient's quality of experience to provide BIS or other DAM monitoring for those patients who are fully paralyzed in ambulatory practice as well as in the inpatient setting. This may be especially useful in patients with an unpredictable need for drugs, such as the obese, the elderly, drug addicts, patients with hypermetabolism, and patients on liver-enzyme-inducing drugs. My routine is to use BIS for TIVA in such patients if they are fully curarized, and also if I am using an inhalational agent and do not want to be above the 1 MAC level. The rule is to avoid continuous BIS values above 60 for 4 min or more and to keep within the range of 45–55.

When DAM is used in noncurarized patients, then the focus is different. These patients will move when anesthesia becomes too light, so DAM should focus on highlighting when patients become anesthetized too deeply following standard dosing. By giving these individual patients less anesthetic and thus speeding their emergence, the average drug consumption and emergence for the whole group of patients will be reduced [49]. Again, this may be especially useful in patients with unpredictable drug requirements (see above) and also during procedures of unpredictable duration and sudden end. In such cases it is hard to titrate the drugs carefully down during the planned end of the procedure, and maintaining an appropriate (not too deep) level at all times is very useful. I use BIS as an adjunct for this purpose in patients with unpredictable dose need during procedures such as laparoscopies and microscopic surgery; the target is to stay in the 50–60 range.

Shall we use laryngeal mask (LMA) for all cases, or do some indications for endotracheal intubation (ET) in ambulatory care remain?

With general anesthesia, an initial period of oxygen supply by mask usually followed by assisted or controlled mask ventilation is mandatory immediately before and just after the loss of consciousness. The question is then, however, how to proceed for maintenance.

The facial mask

This is a valid alternative only if the patient is fasted, as it provides no protection against aspiration. It is also a method that demands full attention and two hands all the time, and with prolonged use it may be cumbersome and strenuous for the anesthetist. There may be problems with maintaining a free airway all the time, and if an oropharyngeal airway is needed this may provoke retching or other reflexes of stress if anesthesia is too low-dosed. If inhalational agents are supplied, the facial mask method will inevitably result in some pollution of the room air. This may be partly counteracted by use of gas suction and evacuation – directly from the airway system, by use of the somewhat cumbersome double-mask, by point-suction close to the patient's mouth, and/or by a high degree of room ventilation. If assisted ventilation has to be used, especially with high pressure, there is a risk of pushing inhalational gas mixture into the esophagus and stomach. Nevertheless the face mask has some advantages: there is no need to use extra equipment with accompanying costs (if disposable) or for cleaning. As no stimulation of the pharynx or larynx is involved, the patient does not need anesthesia for the sake of airway management; thus, if the surgery otherwise allows for low-dose anesthesia, the option for spontaneous ventilation may be available. Also, there is no risk of a sore throat or postoperative airway irritation, as may occur with both LMA and endotracheal tube (ET) placement.

The laryngeal mask (LMA)

Compared with the facial mask, the LMA offers the option of spontaneous breathing and leaves the anesthetist's hands free for other tasks. With a fair and tight fit the free airway is stable, there is minimal leakage of inhalational agents into the surroundings and good control of the gas mixture going into and out of the airways rather than anywhere else (i.e., pollution, patient's stomach). With a tight fit and no need for high-pressure ventilation, the LMA has quite similar characteristics of use as the ET, but the protection afforded against aspiration from a full stomach may be less and the LMA is always potentially more prone to being dislodged, with subsequent problems. This may be a particular problem if surgery is in the mouth or pharynx area, such as adenoidectomy and tonsillectomy. The LMA is also somewhat larger than an ET, and cannot be so readily repositioned for surgical access. Although the LMA stimulates the pharyngeal structures and may traumatize the mucous membranes, there is less need for deep analgesia (or muscle relaxation) and fewer reports of postoperative sore throat and airway problems (i.e., spasm, coughing) than with the ET.

Still in some patients the LMA may be difficult to fit. Then attempts could be made to inflate more air into the LMA cuff, although aiming for the lowest seal pressure. If the seal pressure has to be very high (i.e., more than $45\,cmH_2O$) it may be a sign of improper fit and the high pressure may then cause mucous membrane trauma in those places where the fit is tight. If the fit remains poor after optimal cuff inflation, a larger size of LMA should be attempted. If this also fails, another brand of LMA may be successful, as they are designed slightly differently with a different success rate in individual patients. There have been case reports of stomach ruptures with LMA ventilation, due to a combination of high inspiratory pressures and too much gas leakage into the stomach. For this reason the ProSeal type of LMA may be better as a gastric tube may be inserted through the LMA allowing for gas in the stomach to be evacuated. This may be particularly important during laparoscopy where a 100% empty stomach allows for a better view and better ease of instrumentation. It also serves as a fail-safe mechanism in the very rare occurrence of GI rupture from laparoscopic instrumentation or a high pressure of gas being pushed into the stomach. Although the LMA does not provide a 100% seal of the trachea, it is still argued that it protects the airway very well against modest amounts of mucus or blood from the pharynx area, as the whole entrance of the larynx is covered and protected. However, if the pharynx for some reason (marked bleeding, regurgitation from a full stomach) is "flooded" with fluid, the LMA will not protect fully against airway aspiration, whereas an ET with a properly inflated cuff will.

Endotracheal tube

The benefits of a properly placed ET with inflated cuff are: close to 100% control of all inspiration and expiration in the patient; robustness against the need of high airway pressures; minimal danger of dislocation or aspiration. Classical dogma has been to add muscle relaxants during anesthesia induction to relax the vocal cords and facilitate the ET placement; however, this practice has been challenged by the availability of modern anesthetic agents. With deep levels of anesthesia the vocal cords will be fairly well relaxed and other airway reflexes (coughing) will be abolished, thus the ET can be placed without the need for specific muscle relaxation. However, there are reports of airway damage with this approach, claiming that the use of relaxants makes the intubation more gentle [55]. A more common problem with intubation without relaxants is that the timing of the short intubation trauma may not quite match the peak of the strong analgesic effect, thus a period of severe hypotension may occur before or after the intubation procedure with this approach.

My conclusions

For ambulatory general anesthesia the conventional LMA is the airway device used routinely, after using the facial mask for induction. However, for very short cases, such as dilatation and curettage, myringotomy, and other procedures expected to last for 5–10 min, I use a facial mask throughout. For laparoscopy (gynecologic or gastrointestinal) I use the Pro-Seal type of LMA or another brand and have a gastric tube in position during the surgical procedure. Endotracheal intubation should be used for cases where you anticipate or experience problems with ventilation at normal ventilator pressures, i.e., with a maximum of 20–$30\,cmH_2O$. Before proceeding to endotracheal intubation when an LMA has already been tried, you should check the LMA position at the back of the throat with your finger. Too superficial a level of anesthesia may also be a cause of malpositioning; if the patient bucks or coughs during its insertion, it may not be positioned correctly. A second attempt to position the

LMA after an additional dose of anesthetic may be made. If it leaks despite being sited properly, a larger size LMA may be indicated, as may switching to the ProSeal type or another brand of LMA. Whether a re-usable or a disposable LMA should be used is a question of hygiene and cost; they are similar in terms of ease of insertion and use. It has been shown that proper washing of the LMA removes all infective agents, although you may still find traces of debris that pose a theoretical risk of prion spores. The nondisposable LMAs usually have a guaranteed limit on the number of times they can be used, but in practice this may be exceeded and they are used until they show signs of mechanical wear, which may take more than a year of regular use.

A planned ET may be chosen in selected patients and procedures. Examples are arthritic patients with a stiff rib cage and morbidly obese patients. Some individual decision-making may be involved with the morbidly obese. With a short case (15–30 min), a flat or head-elevated position, and where there is good access to the airways during the procedure, I go for an LMA. Although many obese patients have gastroesophageal regurgitation, this may not be a problem with the LMA if the amounts of fluid are low. Also, using an LMA with a gastric tube will secure the situation. Cases of prolonged laparoscopy (more than 1–2 h) may be done with an ET from the start; the same may apply to procedures on the facial region where access to the airway may be limited during the procedure, such as eye surgery, tonsillectomy, and adenoidectomy. With a skilled surgeon there are many successful reports of using the LMA for adenotonsillectomy, although in a very few cases you may have to change to ET. My favorite for these cases remains the ET, inserted without curare (see Chapter 7). For dental surgery the LMA will often be too cumbersome for the surgeon, and an ET may be more convenient. An oral tube in the corner of the mouth may be used if the surgery is limited to the other side of the oral cavity, and even with bilateral treatment the tube may be moved during the procedure to the other corner. Still, most dental surgeons are happiest if you use a nasal tube, at least for the more extensive and time-consuming procedures. To do so, you should lubricate the nostril and the tube with local anesthetic cream, use topical vasoconstrictor nasal drops, and use more expensive soft-walled tubes to lessen the risk of nasal bleeding. You should examine the patients for signs of ongoing sinusitis or history of frequent sinusitis, as there have been cases of severe sinusitis occurring after nasal intubation beyond 2–3 h.

References

1. Gan TJ, Meyer TA, Apfel CC, et al. Society for Ambulatory Anesthesia guidelines for the management of postoperative nausea and vomiting. *Anesth Analg* 2007;**105**:1615–28, table.

2. Leslie K, Myles PS, Chan MT, et al. Risk factors for severe postoperative nausea and vomiting in a randomized trial of nitrous oxide-based vs nitrous oxide-free anesthesia. *Br J Anaesth* 2008;**101**:498–505.

3. Mathews DM, Gaba V, Zaku B, Neuman GG. Can remifentanil replace nitrous oxide during anesthesia for ambulatory orthopedic surgery with desflurane and fentanyl? *Anesth Analg* 2008;**106**:101–8, table.

4. Handa-Tsutsui F, Kodaka M. Effect of nitrous oxide on propofol requirement during target-controlled infusion for oocyte retrieval. *Int J Obstet Anesth* 2007;**16**:13–16.

5. Gokce BM, Ozkose Z, Tuncer B, et al. Hemodynamic effects, recovery profiles, and costs of remifentanil-based anesthesia with propofol or desflurane for septorhinoplasty. *Saudi Med J* 2007;**28**:358–63.

6. Gozdemir M, Sert H, Yilmaz N, et al. Remifentanil-propofol in vertebral disk operations: hemodynamics and recovery versus desflurane-N(2)O inhalation anesthesia. *Adv Ther* 2007;**24**:622–31.

7. Röhm KD, Riechmann J, Boldt J, et al. Total intravenous anesthesia with propofol and remifentanil is associated with a nearly twofold higher incidence in postanesthetic shivering than desflurane-fentanyl anesthesia. *Med Sci Monit* 2006;**12**:CR452–CR456.

8. Moore JK, Elliott RA, Payne K, et al. The effect of anaesthetic agents on induction, recovery and patient preferences in adult day case surgery: a 7-day follow-up randomized controlled trial. *Eur J Anaesthesiol* 2008;**25**:876–83.

9. Hong JY, Kang YS, Kil HK. Anesthesia for day case excisional breast biopsy: propofol-remifentanil compared with sevoflurane-nitrous oxide. *Eur J Anaesthesiol* 2008;**25**:460–7.

10. Hohlrieder M, Tiefenthaler W, Klaus H, et al. Effect of total intravenous anesthesia and balanced anesthesia on the frequency of coughing during emergence from the anesthesia. *Br J Anaesth* 2007;**99**:587–91.

11. White H, Black RJ, Jones M, Mar Fan GC. Randomized comparison of two anti-emetic strategies in high-risk patients undergoing day-case gynaecological surgery. *Br J Anaesth* 2007;**98**:470–6.

12. Walldén J, Thorn SE, Lovqvist A, et al. The effect of anesthetic technique on early postoperative gastric emptying: comparison of propofol-remifentanil and opioid-free sevoflurane anesthesia. *J Anesth* 2006;**20**:261–7.

13. Stevanovic PD, Petrova G, Miljkovic B, et al. Low fresh gas flow balanced anesthesia versus target controlled intravenous infusion anesthesia in laparoscopic cholecystectomy: a cost-minimization analysis. *Clin Ther* 2008;**30**:1714–25.

14. Yano T, Okubo S, Naruo H, et al. Two cases with past and family history of febrile convulsion developed seizure-like movements during sevoflurane anesthesia. *Anesthesiology* 2008;**109**:571.

15. Grathwohl KW, Black IH, Spinella PC, et al. Total intravenous anesthesia including ketamine versus volatile gas anesthesia for combat-related operative traumatic brain injury. *Anesthesiology* 2008;**109**:44–53.

16. Landoni G, Bignami E, Oliviero F, Zangrillo A. Halogenated anaesthetics and cardiac protection in cardiac and non-cardiac anesthesia. *Ann Card Anaesth* 2009;**12**:4–9.

17. Kim JY, Chang YJ, Lee JY, et al. Post-induction alfentanil reduces sevoflurane-associated emergence agitation in children undergoing an adenotonsillectomy. *Acta Anaesthesiol Scand* 2009;**53**:678–81.

18. Lee JS, Gonzalez ML, Chuang SK, Perrott DH. Comparison of methohexital and propofol use in ambulatory procedures in oral and maxillofacial surgery. *J Oral Maxillofac Surg* 2008;**66**:1996–2003.

19. Raeder JC, Stenseth LB. Ketamine: a new look at an old drug. *Curr Opin Anaesthesiol* 2000;**13**:463–8.

20. Strayer RJ, Nelson LS. Adverse events associated with ketamine for procedural sedation in adults. *Am J Emerg Med* 2008;**26**:985–1028.

21. Friedberg BL. Propofol-ketamine technique. *Aesthetic Plast Surg* 1993;**17**:297–300.

22. Friedberg BL. Propofol ketamine anesthesia for cosmetic surgery in the office suite. *Int Anesthesiol Clin* 2003;**41**:39–50.

23. Rapeport DA, Martyr JW, Wang LP. The use of "ketofol" (ketamine-propofol admixture) infusion in conjunction with regional anesthesia. *Anaesth Intensive Care* 2009;**37**:121–3.

24. Messenger DW, Murray HE, Dungey PE, et al. Subdissociative-dose ketamine versus fentanyl for analgesia during propofol procedural sedation: a randomized clinical trial. *Acad Emerg Med* 2008;**15**:877–86.

25. Aouad MT, Moussa AR, Dagher CM, et al. Addition of ketamine to propofol for initiation of procedural anesthesia in children reduces propofol consumption and preserves hemodynamic stability. *Acta Anaesthesiol Scand* 2008;**52**:561–5.

26. Goel S, Bhardwaj N, Jain K. Efficacy of ketamine and midazolam as co-induction agents with propofol for laryngeal mask insertion in children. *Paediatr Anaesth* 2008;**18**:628–34.

27. Slavik VC, Zed PJ. Combination ketamine and propofol for procedural sedation and analgesia. *Pharmacotherapy* 2007;**27**:1588–98.

28. De Kock MF, Lavand'homme PM. The clinical role of NMDA receptor antagonists for the treatment of postoperative pain. *Best Pract Res Clin Anaesthesiol* 2007;**21**:85–98.

29. Gravningsbråten R, Nicklasson B, Raeder J. Safety of laryngeal mask airway and short-stay practice in office-based adenotonsillectomy. *Acta Anaesthesiol Scand* 2009;**53**:218–22.

30. Paek CM, Yi JW, Lee BJ, Kang JM. No supplemental muscle relaxants are required during propofol and remifentanil total intravenous anesthesia for laparoscopic pelvic surgery. *J Laparoendosc Adv Surg Tech A* 2009;**19**:33–7.

31. Baillard C, Adnet F, Borron SW, et al. Tracheal intubation in routine practice with and without muscular relaxation: an observational study. *Eur J Anaesthesiol* 2005;**22**:672–7.

32. Mencke T, Echternach M, Plinkert PK, et al. Does the timing of tracheal intubation based on neuromuscular monitoring decrease laryngeal injury? A randomized, prospective, controlled trial. *Anesth Analg* 2006;**102**:306–12.

33. Devereaux PJ, Yang H, Yusuf S, et al. Effects of extended-release metoprolol succinate in patients undergoing non-cardiac surgery (POISE trial): a randomised controlled trial. *Lancet* 2008;**371**:1839–47.

34. Bilotta F, Lam AM, Doronzio A, et al. Esmolol blunts postoperative hemodynamic changes after propofol-remifentanil total intravenous fast-track neuroanesthesia for intracranial surgery. *J Clin Anesth* 2008;**20**:426–30.

35. Collard V, Mistraletti G, Taqi A, et al. Intraoperative esmolol infusion in the absence of opioids spares postoperative fentanyl in patients undergoing ambulatory laparoscopic cholecystectomy. *Anesth Analg* 2007;**105**:1255–62, table.

36. Leslie K, Clavisi O, Hargrove J. Target-controlled infusion versus manually controlled infusion of propofol for general anesthesia or sedation in adults. *Cochrane Database Syst Rev* 2008;CD006059.

37. Bressan N, Castro A, Braga C, et al. Automation in anesthesia: computer controlled propofol infusion and data acquisition. *Conf Proc IEEE Eng Med Biol Soc* 2008;**2008**:5543–7.

38. De Smet T, Struys MM, Neckebroek MM, et al. The accuracy and clinical feasibility of a new Bayesian-based closed-loop control system for propofol administration using the bispectral index as a controlled variable. *Anesth Analg* 2008;**107**:1200–10.

39. Liu N, Chazot T, Trillat B, et al. Feasibility of closed-loop titration of propofol guided by the bispectral index for general anesthesia induction: a prospective randomized study. *Eur J Anaesthesiol* 2006;**23**:465–9.

40. Sawaguchi Y, Furutani E, Shirakami G, et al. A model-predictive hypnosis control system under total intravenous anesthesia. *IEEE Trans Biomed Eng* 2008;**55**:874–87.

41. Carollo DS, Nossaman BD, Ramadhyani U. Dexmedetomidine: a review of clinical applications. *Curr Opin Anaesthesiol* 2008;**21**:457–61.

42. Zeyneloglu P, Pirat A, Candan S, et al. Dexmedetomidine causes prolonged recovery when compared with midazolam/fentanyl combination in outpatient shock wave lithotripsy. *Eur J Anaesthesiol* 2008;**25**:961–7.

43. Salman N, Uzun S, Coskun F, et al. Dexmedetomidine as a substitute for remifentanil in ambulatory gynecologic laparoscopic surgery. *Saudi Med J* 2009;**30**:77–81.

44. Soltesz S, Silomon M, Graf G, et al. Effect of a 0.5% dilution of propofol on pain on injection during induction of anesthesia in children. *Anesthesiology* 2007;**106**:80–4.

45. Silvestri GA, Vincent BD, Wahidi MM, et al. A phase 3, randomized, double-blind study to assess the efficacy and safety of fospropofol disodium injection for moderate sedation in patients undergoing flexible bronchoscopy. *Chest* 2009;**135**:41–7.

46. Upton RN, Martinez AM, Grant C. Comparison of the sedative properties of CNS 7056, midazolam, and propofol in sheep. *Br J Anaesth* 2009;**103**:848–57.

47. Einarsson SG, Cerne A, Bengtsson A, et al. Respiration during emergence from anesthesia with desflurane/N_2O vs. desflurane/air for gynaecological

laparoscopy. *Acta Anaesthesiol Scand* 1998;**42**:1192–8.

48. Cheong KF, Low TC. Propofol and postanesthetic shivering. *Anaesthesia* 1995;**50**:550–2.

49. White PF. Use of cerebral monitoring during anesthesia: effect on recovery profile. *Best Pract Res Clin Anaesthesiol* 2006;**20**:181–9.

50. Gjerstad AC, Storm H, Hagen R, et al. Skin conductance or entropy for detection of non-noxious stimulation during different clinical levels of sedation. *Acta Anaesthesiol Scand* 2007;**51**:1–7.

51. Hoymork SC, Hval K, Jensen EW, Raeder J. Can the cerebral state monitor replace the bispectral index in monitoring hypnotic effect during propofol/remifentanil anesthesia? *Acta Anaesthesiol Scand* 2007;**51**:210–16.

52. Ekman A, Lindholm ML, Lennmarken C, Sandin R. Reduction in the incidence of awareness using BIS monitoring. *Acta Anaesthesiol Scand* 2004;**48**:20–6.

53. Myles PS, Leslie K, McNeil J, et al. Bispectral index monitoring to prevent awareness during anesthesia: the B-Aware randomised controlled trial. *Lancet* 2004;**363**:1757–63.

54. Alpiger S, Helbo-Hansen HS, Vach W, Ording H. Efficacy of the A-line AEP monitor as a tool for predicting successful insertion of a laryngeal mask during sevoflurane anesthesia. *Acta Anaesthesiol Scand* 2004;**48**:888–93.

55. Combes X, Andriamifidy L, Dufresne, et al. Comparison of two induction regimes using or not using muscle relaxant: impact on postoperative upper airway discomfort. *Br J Anaesth* 2007;**99**:276–81.

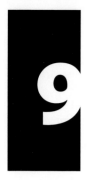

9 Success criteria and future of ambulatory anesthesia

Success criteria [1]

The success of ambulatory anesthesia and surgery may be measured in the following different areas:

- Patient safety: mortality and morbidity
- Patient quality
- Cost-efficiency
- Satisfaction of employees and employers
- Role in education, training, and research.

These topics are covered broadly in many textbooks of ambulatory surgery and selected important issues are discussed here.

Patient safety

As mentioned previously there is zero tolerance for mortality in ambulatory care; patients with a predicted risk of dying from their surgery or anesthesia should be planned as inpatients. The tolerance for permanent disability due to anesthesia is also zero, whereas a very small risk of surgical failure or chronic pain from certain procedures may be calculated. It is essential that every unit has a system for collecting data on cases that have a bad outcome, whether through reports to health authorities, insurance companies, or through other dedicated systems designed for the local circumstances.

Patient quality

All units should have a system for collecting quality data from all patients. This is best achieved as a daily routine for all patients or as a regular and random check on selected patients. Quality can be quantified in terms of patient satisfaction with the following issues:

- Preoperative waiting time
- Preoperative information
- Preoperative hours spent and travelling logistics (including parking), for both preoperative visits and on the day of surgery
- Low risk of being canceled on the day of surgery
- The feeling of being involved in decision-making with regards to surgery and type of anesthesia
- Friendliness and professional attitude of the personnel at all phases

- The location, design, and practical aspects of the building
- The surgical result: as expected? no side-effects? short rehabilitation?
- Anesthesiologic quality: no awareness, minimal anxiety, pleasant induction, pleasant loco-regional method (if used), no postoperative nausea or vomiting, minimal pain, minimal dizziness or other side-effects
- No need for unanticipated overnight stay in a hospital
- Postoperative information
- Quality of follow-up from the unit (phone call? questionnaire?)
- Home travel
- Function and well-being at home; burden on relatives/friends?
- Need for unanticipated contact with health personnel and/or re-admission?
- Final outcome
- Patient's overall satisfaction

Cost-efficiency

Cost-efficiency is determined by many local issues, with some or all from the following list:

- Rate of cancelation of planned procedures
- Time of start of first operation in the morning
- Length of surgery and anesthesia for selected procedures
- Time delay from the end of one procedure to the start of the next in a particular theater
- Time of the end of the last procedure of the day. (Ending late unplanned is suboptimal as this requires extra payment and may be a source of personnel dissatisfaction)
- Prolonged recovery stay or prolonged stay in the unit
- Extra postoperative work or costs linked with complications or side-effects
- Unplanned reoperation
- Unplanned discharge directly to inpatient care instead of going home
- Unplanned readmission to hospital

Also other obvious economic issues will be important here, such as salary agreements, number of employees, qualification of employees (level of salary), use of equipment, disposables, and drugs, etc.

Satisfaction of employees and employers, and role in education, training, and research

This issue is sometimes forgotten, but is a very important benchmark of success. Not all units have a role in education, training, or research, but those that do must be evaluated for these achievements as well. It must also be recognized that success in education, training, and research may interfere with the narrow scope of cost-efficiency.

The satisfaction of employees may be evaluated based on the popularity of newly available positions in the unit, the rate at which employees resign, and also the rate of sick leave. Questionnaires on satisfaction and employee talks should be organized regularly. A program of education, meetings, and congress participation and traveling to see other units may also be very rewarding for employee satisfaction and thus other aspects of unit quality.

Some future aspects of ambulatory surgery and anesthesia

In the future we may expect developments in ambulatory anesthesia and surgery in terms of drugs, equipment, surgical procedures, patient population, and organization.

The successful development of an esterase-degraded propofol analog sleeping agent may further improve the speed of emergence after intravenous anesthesia. A more short-acting benzodiazepine drug is presently under development and may result in renewed interest in using benzodiazepine as the major hypnotic for TIVA anesthesia. Xenon is a promising, although still very expensive and probably somewhat emetogenic, inhalational agent with a rapid on–off effect, a minor influence on circulation and respiration, and no pollution problems. New, highly efficient and rapidly acting neuromuscular blocking reversal agents are presently being tested on patients.

With local anesthesia we hope for a breakthrough in the research for safe, slow-release formulations that provide a local anesthetic effect for days after a single injection. This would be an important asset in the field of postoperative pain relief, where we remain in need of better drugs and methods. There are a lot of new and interesting analgesic drug principles in the pipeline, mainly based on known mediators of pain in the periphery and spinal cord.

For PONV prophylaxis and treatment, the NK1 antagonists seem to be a new and important drug principle, adding to those already available for multimodal options.

In terms of monitoring there may be an option to introduce more sophisticated non-invasive monitoring of cardiovascular and respiratory function. There are already numerous ongoing attempts to realize the concepts of anesthetic-depth monitoring. An important breakthrough here will occur once we can achieve online monitoring of surgical stress (in addition to sleep), so as to better individualize the dosing of analgesic drugs during general anesthesia. Better TCI algorithms may help us to improve drug dosing, and research into end-tidal technology for measuring plasma propofol and other drugs is very interesting.

We are sure to see further developments in the production of less expensive and less bulky equipment, as well as in wireless technology, which will improve the working environment in the operating theater and also facilitate the establishment of monitoring in the preoperative holding area, and enable smooth transition of the patient with full monitoring to the PACU after a procedure.

Internet technology will spread further, improving the availability of every patient's health record and providing better exchange of information between health care providers and the patient, both before and after the procedure. In terms of organization, we have already developed more office-based surgery and anesthesia. This will probably be enhanced as drugs and equipment improve, although we will always have to keep a close watch that appropriate standards of care are being applied when we move out of the hospital and no longer have all its attendant backup facilities readily to hand.

We should expect surgery to become increasingly noninvasive, moving from open surgical fields toward more and more endoscopy. For instance, a hip prosthesis may be done using endoscopic equipment. Robotic surgery and surgery with ongoing imaging are both evolving, as is invasive radiology for which some procedures may be best done in ambulatory units.

In the western world, we will see more patients who are obese and more elderly patients. Patients will increasingly have access to the internet and many will have a good level of knowledge and will specify demands for their safety and quality of ambulatory care. Society's demands for quality assurance and documentation are on the increase.

We will see growth of ambulatory care into hospitals and geographic areas that will catch up with that provided in pioneering institutions. From a global perspective, we should also expect increased interest in ambulatory care in less developed parts of the world.

Reference

1. Lemos P, Regalado AM. Patient outcomes and clinical indicators for ambulatory surgery. In: Lemos P, Jarrett P, Philip B, eds. *Day Surgery – Development and Practice*, London: IAAS, 2006: 257–80.

Index